T0355158

Rethinking Suicide

Rethinking Suicide

Why Prevention Fails, and
How We Can Do Better

CRAIG J. BRYAN

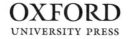

OXFORD
UNIVERSITY PRESS

OXFORD
UNIVERSITY PRESS

Oxford University Press is a department of the University of Oxford. It furthers
the University's objective of excellence in research, scholarship, and education
by publishing worldwide. Oxford is a registered trade mark of Oxford University
Press in the UK and certain other countries.

Published in the United States of America by Oxford University Press
198 Madison Avenue, New York, NY 10016, United States of America.

Library of Congress Cataloging-in-Publication Data
Names: Bryan, Craig J., author.
Title: Rethinking suicide : why prevention fails, and how we can do better / Craig J. Bryan.
Description: New York : Oxford University Press, 2022. |
Includes bibliographical references and index.
Identifiers: LCCN 2021005698 | ISBN 9780190050634 (hardback) |
ISBN 9780190050658 (epub) | ISBN 9780197577882
Subjects: LCSH: Soldiers–Suicidal behavior. |
Suicide–Psychological aspects. | War–Psychological aspects.
Classification: LCC HV6545.7 .B79 2021 | DDC 362.28088/355–dc23
LC record available at https://lccn.loc.gov/2021005698

DOI: 10.1093/med-psych/9780190050634.001.0001

5 7 9 8 6

Printed by Sheridan Books, Inc., United States of America

For Mom, Dad, Renee, and AnnaBelle

Contents

Introduction

I'm often asked which came first: researching suicide or joining the military. The question is hard to answer because, on the one hand, suicide has been of interest to me, at least to some degree, as far back as high school. On the other hand, it wasn't until I was deployed to Iraq in 2009—where I stood over the bodies of service members who had died of self-inflicted gunshot wounds—that my commitment to researching and preventing suicide was cemented.

The U.S. invasion of Iraq, also known as Operation Iraqi Freedom, began on Thursday, March 20, 2003, during my second semester of graduate school. Because Thursdays were class days in our graduate program, all of the clinical graduate students were on campus that day. As first-year students, my classmates and I were enrolled in Interpersonal Psychotherapy that semester, which was taught back then by David Kopplin. At the start of class, Dr. Kopplin said he wanted to have a brief discussion about world events before getting into the planned topics for the day. I remember Dr. Kopplin's concern that, as a nation, we were not talking with enough depth about the consequences of armed conflict, especially the psychological costs of war. A very small number of men and women, he feared, would bear the disproportionate weight of this cost. As clinical psychologists, he added, we would play an important role in helping these men and women to deal with these costs, potentially for the rest of their lives.

On the morning of March 23, 2003, I had no reason to suspect that I would ever join the military. To be honest, I don't think I was even aware that psychologists served in the military. Nonetheless, on March 28, 2005, almost two years to the day after that conversation in Dr. Kopplin's class, I raised my right hand in an Air Force recruiting station in Dallas, Texas, and took the Oath of Commissioned Officers, becoming a military officer and Air Force psychologist. Joining the military was, admittedly, a direction that few people—including myself—would have ever predicted for me; I certainly wasn't the "military type." For many years, when friends and family would ask me why I chose to pursue this unexpected path, I couldn't really explain it very well; I just felt like I *had* to do it. Today, nearly a decade and a half later and with the benefit of hindsight, I think the idea of joining the military was first planted by Dr. Kopplin on March 23, 2003, when he delayed the start of our class to talk about the consequences of war. That seed was subsequently watered and nourished by David Rudd, who was the Director of Clinical Training when I was a graduate student and would become a key mentor over the course of my career. David had served as an Army psychologist during the first Persian Gulf War, and encouraged me over the course of my graduate training to consider military service as a professional path. *It's meaningful work*, David repeatedly told me during my years as a student; *there's nothing else like it.*

I served on active duty as a psychologist for just over four years—from 2005 to 2009—at Lackland Air Force Base in San Antonio, Texas, although the final six months of my active duty service were spent at Joint Base Balad, Iraq.[1] I arrived in Iraq in late February 2009 with the primary mission of running the Traumatic Brain Injury Clinic attached to the Air Force Theater Hospital, a forward-deployed military hospital that was equivalent to a Level-I trauma center in the United States.[2] In this role, I conducted neurocognitive assessments and provided treatment for U.S. military personnel and coalition forces who had sustained head injuries. On top of these responsibilities, my duties included providing consultation to the medical and surgical staff working in the hospital and providing psychological treatment to the 20,000-plus military personnel stationed on the base. Although my job in Iraq was similar in many respects to my job in the United States—conducting diagnostic assessments, providing psychological treatment, consulting with commanders—the context of Iraq was very different, to say the least. In the United States, for instance, when I talked with service members about deployment-related trauma, we were typically talking about events that had happened years before. In Iraq, however, when I talked with service members about these same topics and issues, we often were talking about events that had happened only a few days, or even mere hours, before.

In Iraq, I came face to face with trauma and the brutality of suicide in a way I had not experienced before. Among deployed military personnel, suicides are almost exclusively the result of self-inflicted gunshot wound, owing to the fact that deployed military personnel have very easy access to loaded firearms pretty much all the time. When I was in Iraq, deceased service members would sometimes be received by our hospital and held temporarily, hooked up to various life support devices to preserve organ functioning while awaiting transport back to the United States. Once home, those who had volunteered as organ donors were taken to the operating room for transplant surgery. We followed these procedures for all deceased service members, regardless of the manner of death, including suicide decedents. Suicide decedents tended to have a different effect on us, though. When a suicide decedent was in the hospital, the mood and climate seemed to shift. It wasn't a dramatic change, but it was noticeable; something you "felt" more than observed. I remember one day during lunch with a small group of hospital staff, someone asked if the deceased service member who had arrived earlier that day "was a suicide." No one in the group was sure, but someone asked why she wanted to know. "No reason," she answered. "It just feels like suicide." After lunch, we learned that she was right: The deceased service member who had arrived that morning had died by suicide.

During another week of my deployment, four service members who had died by suicide were in the hospital at the same time. This was unusual; during a typical week there would be no suicide decedents in the hospital. When we *did* have suicide decedents in the hospital, there were usually only one or two, at most, in the intensive care unit at the same time. During that particular week, however, it just so happened that the hospital census was low, meaning that we had very few patients with severe injuries. By sheer coincidence, a sandstorm blew in that same week. The sandstorm wasn't particularly severe, but it was bad enough that lower priority flights were halted.[3] The combination of low patient census and suboptimal flight conditions resulted in an unusually long stay for these four service members—several days rather than the day or less that was more common. Because of the low census, all four suicide decedents were placed side by side in the intensive care unit so it was easier to monitor and care for them. After a few days with us, I remember standing at the foot of one of the center beds, looking back and forth across all four men, and being struck by the seeming juxtaposition of life and death that each one represented. On the one hand, all four men were very much dead. On the other hand, their organs were still "alive" because we were pumping blood and oxygen through their veins and closely watching the functioning of their various biological systems. Their chests rose and fell and their heart monitors chirped with regularity, almost as if they were all just quietly taking naps at the same time.

I also remember the savage nature of their injuries. All four men had died of self-inflicted gunshot wounds to the head. Emergency medicine, trauma, and surgical staff are (tragically) all too well-acquainted with these types of injuries, but as a psychologist, this was my first face-to-face encounter with the ruthlessness of suicide. Emergency department staff and trauma surgeons don't page the on-call psychologist or psychiatrist when a patient dies as a result of their suicidal behavior; they only call us when a patient survives. Standing over the bodies of those four service members, I remember feeling a mixture of sadness about their deaths, frustration that I couldn't do anything to undo their problems or fix things for them, and anger that I never had the opportunity to help them. I wondered about who they were and what they had done in their lives. Were they married or partnered? Did they have any children? Where were they from and what did they enjoy doing? I also wondered what had happened on the day they died. Why did they pull the trigger on that particular day at that particular time? What had changed for them as compared to the previous day, week, and month? What if the circumstances had been different? My understanding of suicide was changed forever by this experience, and I came to realize that the prevailing model for suicide prevention was limited by survival bias, a logical error wherein we focus on the people or things that survive some selection process while overlooking those who did not.

I first learned about survival bias from the story of Abraham Wald, a Jewish mathematician who emigrated to the United States during World War II to escape Nazi oppression and eventually played a pivotal role in saving the lives of countless military aviators. During World War II, U.S. planes launched from Britain often returned from missions riddled with bullet holes resulting from antiaircraft fire. These were the lucky ones; many planes did not return at all. To minimize these losses, the military decided to add more armor to their planes, thereby providing greater protection from antiaircraft fire. The problem was that extra armor increased the plane's weight, necessitating more fuel to fly the same distance or the removal of bombs and ammunition to offset that weight. To balance the need for increased protection without adding too much weight, military leaders decided to concentrate the armor in the most vulnerable sections of the planes rather than covering the entire plan with extra armor. But which sections of the planes should they focus on? The Navy conducted a study to answer this question. In that study, researchers modeled the average density of bullet holes observed among returning planes; they found that the average number of bullet holes per square foot was not uniform across returning planes. The fuselage, for instance, tended to have more bullet holes per square foot than the engines. Based on these results, the military concluded that it would be more effective to add extra armor to the fuselage than to the engines, as this was clearly the section of the plane that was sustaining the greatest amount of damage. In the end, however, the military did the exact opposite: they added extra armor to the engines and to the other sections of the plane that had the *fewest*, not the most, bullet holes.

This change was influenced by Wald, who identified a critical error in the reasoning of the military officers charged with finding a solution that could reduce the number of downed planes. At the outset of the Navy's study, the only planes included were those that made it back from a mission—the survivors. The planes that were shot down in enemy airspace or did not make it back to base were not included because they were "missing"—they did not survive and were therefore "invisible" to the researchers. Wald recognized the error this introduced into the military's logic—this survival bias—and asked a somewhat different question: Why do some sections of the plane have fewer bullet holes than others? Wald based this question on the assumption that all sections of the plane were equally vulnerable to antiaircraft fire. All of the sections of a plane, therefore, should have had a similar number of bullet holes, but they didn't. Wald realized that the "missing" bullet holes were on the planes that didn't make it back. The reason the engines on the surviving planes had fewer bullet holes per square foot wasn't because this was where the planes were *least* vulnerable; it was because this was where the planes were *most* vulnerable. If a plane's engine was shot and damaged, it was much more likely to lose the power and fuel needed to return home. If a plane's fuselage was shot and damaged, however, there was still a chance that the plane could make it back. If the Navy wanted to increase the number of planes and the number of people who returned, they needed to think about what could not be seen rather than what was sitting in front of them.

Wald convinced the Navy to see things from this perspective, and the recommendation was put into place: extra armor was concentrated in the engine sections instead of the fuselage. The strategy worked. Fewer planes were shot down, and many lives were saved. The strategy did not save every plane and every life, of course, but it made a big difference. Without Wald's intervention, the military almost certainly would have placed extra armor on plane fuselage sections, and they almost certainly would have seen little to no change in survival rates despite seeing fewer bullet holes in the up-armored sections of the newly returned planes. Perhaps the smaller number of bullet holes in the armored sections of returning planes would have led them to conclude that the extra armor worked, although the unchanged number of planes being shot down might have confused them. If the planes have fewer bullet holes, they might have wondered, then why aren't more returning home? Maybe they would have added even more armor to those same sections, hoping that the added protection would do the trick, but that would have ultimately proven futile. This cycle of armoring up the wrong sections of the plane without any change in outcome would have lasted, to the befuddlement and confusion of researchers, pilots, officers, and everyone else involved, unable to realize that the application of a good intervention can nonetheless result in failure if it's based on a faulty assumption.

We currently face a similar situation with respect to suicide in the United States. Over the past two decades, the U.S. suicide rate has steadily increased despite expanded efforts to reverse this trend, to the frustration of researchers, clinicians, family members, and many others. Why do suicide rates continue to rise despite our best efforts? Why aren't we better at this? What are we doing wrong?

This book seeks answers to these questions. Central to this effort is the assumption that suicide is best understood as a "wicked problem," a concept described in a 1973 paper by Horst Rittel and Melvin Webber meant to characterize social policy problems, which are notoriously difficult to solve. Wicked problems are distinguished from conventional problems by their high level of complexity, rendering them especially tricky to solve. This inherent complexity results in constant change, which reduces the probability that any particular strategy will fully address the problem. To this end, wicked problems cannot be definitively solved or completely eliminated— an especially unsettling and uncomfortable perspective when applied to a problem such as suicide. Solutions to wicked problems, therefore, cannot be "right" or "wrong," although some solutions may be relatively better or worse than others. This means there is no "one thing" we can do to prevent suicide, and there probably isn't a "best" thing or "most important" thing that we can do, either.

This is not to say, however, that nothing can be done to prevent suicide. As will be discussed in this book, several strategies are very clearly better than others at preventing suicide, although none of these strategies alone is enough to eliminate suicide completely. We must, therefore, abandon a solution-oriented perspective, which assumes that a "right" or "best" solution exists, and adopt a process-oriented approach instead, wherein we recognize that any given strategy that reduces suicide under certain conditions may nonetheless have very little effect—or maybe even make things worse— under other conditions. Furthermore, we need to realize that even when we have identified and employed one or more strategies that prevent suicides, additional strategies will almost certainly be needed in the future to maintain these initial gains and adapt to the ever-changing nature of suicide.

Consistent with the perspective of suicide as a wicked problem, I will argue in this book that we need to replace our solution-based approach to suicide prevention with a process-based approach focused on creating and building lives worth living. I will further argue that a process-based approach would include the following key features: (1) becoming comfortable with what we don't know; (2) embracing the inherent complexity of suicide; (3) moving beyond a mental-illness-based model of suicide; (4) recognizing the importance of context; (5) being willing to change what we do even when it's uncomfortable or inconvenient; and (6) attending to quality-of-life issues and social factors that influence the perceived value of living. Keeping people alive is certainly a worthy goal, but if we do not take the time to create and build lives that are worth living, our efforts will ultimately fail.

This book begins with a critique of contemporary suicide prevention efforts. In Chapter 1, I consider how our collective discomfort with the many things that we don't know about suicide constrains innovative thinking about suicide. In Chapter 2, I critically evaluate the central role of mental illness and argue that the predominance of this perspective reflects confirmation bias, which is the tendency to search for and interpret information in a way that supports our beliefs and assumptions. Finally, in Chapter 3, I discuss how the mental illness model of suicide has led us to place more faith than may be warranted in concepts such as suicide "warning signs" and suicide-risk screening tools, which are notoriously unreliable indicators of emerging suicidal behaviors because they do not sufficiently reflect the inherently dynamic and ever-changing nature of suicide risk.

I then introduce several alternative perspectives that could improve suicide prevention efforts. First, in Chapter 4, I provide an overview of newer thinking about how suicide risk fluctuates over time using concepts informed by mathematics, which provides a useful model for understanding why and how suicide emerges in different ways for different people at different times. I focus in particular on the implications of this perspective for understanding suicides that emerge suddenly or "out of the blue" without much advance notice or warning signs. Next, in Chapter 5, I argue that suicide can be more usefully understood as a consequence of decision-making processes that are vulnerable to environment and social influence rather than a consequence of internal states or traits such as mental illness.

In the final chapters, I discuss the implications of these ideas for suicide prevention, and I outline several processes that could, in combination, obtain better results. In Chapter 6, I focus on the mental healthcare system, which has been surprisingly slow to adopt the treatments and interventions that are most likely to reduce the probability that someone will attempt suicide. Treatment-focused strategies, however, are not enough. In Chapter 7, I therefore argue for a potentially high-impact but underutilized strategy: restricting or limiting access to highly lethal methods for suicide, especially firearms. Finally, in Chapter 8, I argue that suicide prevention is more than just stopping people from dying; it's also about reducing the social conditions that negatively affect quality of life while strengthening the conditions that promote and foster meaningful lives that are worth living.

Ultimately, my aim with this book is to challenge some of our core assumptions about suicide and typical practices that may not be so helpful or useful after all, and to present alternative perspectives that implicate different approaches that may work better than prevailing methods. These alternative perspectives have been heavily influenced by the many suicidal individuals who have shared their experiences, trials, and triumphs with me over the years. Listening to their stories and voices has helped me to consider angles and ideas that may not have been readily accessible or recognizable, and helped me to see suicide as a wicked problem that cannot be solved using traditional assumptions and approaches.

The perspective gained from these voices has proven to be invaluable, but none more so than the perspective gained from those four Soldiers in Iraq over whom I stood just over a decade ago. As I have reflected upon that moment over the years that have since passed, I am reminded of a saying commonly inscribed on the walls and doors of anatomical theaters, pathology labs, autopsy rooms, and gross anatomy instruction rooms in medical schools all around the world: *This is the place where death delights to help the living.* I can't remember when or where I first stumbled across this saying, but to me the proverb represents so many of the personal and professional experiences that have guided my work as a clinician and researcher. "When that person died," Jared Rich notes in a 2009 essay reflecting upon this saying, "it was one life lost, but in their death, they have given life to countless other people, and they have done that through us." My hope is that, through this book, the lessons I learned from those four men in Iraq, and so many others, will give life to others.

1

On the Merits of Productive Stupidity

When I joined the Air Force in 2005, hostilities in Iraq were escalating, resulting in more frequent and longer deployments for just about everyone serving in the military, including psychologists. Soon thereafter, the suicide rate among military personnel also started to rise, especially in the Army and Marine Corps. During the first few years of that upward trend, the general sense was that the military was just having a few "bad years." In 2008, however, the age- and gender-adjusted Army and Marine suicide rates surpassed the U.S. general population rate.[1] By the time I deployed to Iraq in February 2009, the military suicide rate had been rising steadily for three consecutive years; the initial assumption that we were simply experiencing a few bad years had dissolved, and an uncomfortable recognition that we had a clear problem on our hands had taken hold.

During the four years of my active duty military service, I recall there being a general sense of anxiety and urgency about this issue, both within the military community and among the public as a whole. Nearly a decade later, suicide rates remain elevated across all four branches of the military, but the sense of urgency that once gripped us has all but vanished, seemingly replaced by a shared sense of resignation over this "new normal." I suppose that this growing sense of indifference isn't surprising when one considers how many hundreds of millions of dollars have been invested in military suicide prevention efforts with little to no benefit. This is not to say that *nothing* has been accomplished in the past decade; on the contrary, military- and VA-sponsored research has led to several critical advances in our understanding of suicide, especially in the areas of suicide risk assessment and treatment. Despite these advances, however, military suicide rates have yet to come back down, an unpleasant reality that has fueled considerable frustration.

Seeking to Understand Military Suicide: An Early Lesson

Because military suicides initially started to rise in the years after the start of military operations in Afghanistan and Iraq, an early hypothesis was that the excess of suicides were caused by increasing deployments. The rationale underlying this relationship was largely (though not entirely) influenced by the widely held perspective that suicide is caused by or results from mental illness. Deployments were known to increase rates of mental illness, especially post-traumatic stress disorder (PTSD), substance use disorders, and depression. These mental illnesses were, in turn, assumed to cause suicide because, as we all know, suicide is caused by or results from mental illness. This explanation was quickly embraced by many people—specialists and laypersons alike—for a number of reasons, including its simplicity and intuitiveness.

For many researchers and mental health professionals like me, this explanation was further bolstered by the 2007 publication of the book, *Why People Die by Suicide*, by Thomas Joiner, a clinical psychologist who is one of the world's most prominent and influential suicide researchers. In his book, Joiner laid out a new theory of suicide that he had been developing and researching over many years, namely, the *interpersonal-psychological theory*. According to this theory, dying by suicide (or making a nearly lethal suicide attempt) requires the combination of suicidal *desire* (in other words, wanting to die by suicide) and suicidal *capability* (possessing the ability to attempt suicide). Suicidal desire and suicidal capability are both necessary for suicide, but neither is sufficient on its own. In other words, wanting to kill oneself is not enough to die by suicide; one must also be able to do it. Likewise, possessing the ability to attempt suicide is not enough; one must also want to die.

The requirement for having both desire and capability provides a simple and easy-to-understand explanation for why suicidal behavior occurs so infrequently, even among individuals who are thinking about suicide. According to Substance Abuse and Mental Health Service Administration data, approximately 10.6 million adults had serious thoughts about suicide, 1.4 million made a suicide attempt, and 40,000 died by suicide in 2017.[2] This means that, out of 1,000 U.S. adults who have serious thoughts about suicide each year, 868 do *not* attempt suicide and 997 do *not* die by suicide. According to the interpersonal-psychological theory, the many, many people who think about suicide but who do not attempt or die by suicide may desire suicide, but probably do not possess the ability to act upon this desire.

The interpersonal-psychological theory further posits that suicidal capability involves the combination of a diminished fear of death and heightened pain tolerance. Both of these variables—fearlessness and pain tolerance—can be acquired over time through repeated exposure to painful and provocative experiences such as aggression, violence, trauma, and physical injury, which were believed to be especially central. This is not the only way that fearlessness and pain tolerance can develop, but this particular explanation—that the capability for suicide could develop over time as the result of exposure to adverse life experiences characterized by violence and aggression—was especially attractive to many of us who worked with (and for) the military, because it aligned with military cultural values such as strength, courage, and mental toughness. The interpersonal-psychological theory, therefore, provided a straightforward explanation for understanding why and how deployments could contribute to rising suicide rates among military personnel.

As with many other contemporary suicide researchers, my own work has been heavily influenced by the interpersonal-psychological theory. In one of my earliest research studies, for example, I collected self-report data from Air Force personnel who had recently graduated from basic training. In that study, we found that Airmen who reported higher levels of fearlessness tended to have more severe suicide risk histories, just as the interpersonal-psychological theory proposes. We also found that fearlessness scores were higher than the scores previously reported among civilians who had made multiple suicide attempts. This was an especially compelling finding to many of us, because individuals who have attempted suicide multiple times tend to report high levels of fearlessness about death and are much more likely to attempt suicide again, as compared to individuals who have never attempted suicide or who have attempted suicide only once. Our finding, therefore, suggested that military personnel, even those who were very young and had no history of deployment, were less afraid of death than civilians who had repeatedly attempted suicide. When we later found similar results in a separate sample of deployed military personnel, we became increasingly confident in the conclusion that military personnel possessed greater suicidal capability. This characteristic or trait made it easier for them to attempt suicide.

Another facet of the interpersonal-psychological theory that we tested early in my research career was the hypothesis that suicidal capability could be acquired via exposure to violence, aggression, trauma, and other painful and provocative experiences. To test this notion, we conducted two separate analyses designed to examine how combat exposure was related to fearlessness about death. In the first study, we found a positive correlation: military personnel who reported more severe combat exposure also reported more fearlessness about death. In the second study, we conducted a more sophisticated analysis designed to determine whether various types of deployment experiences were correlated to various degrees with fearlessness about death. Our results indicated that experiences characterized by high levels of violence and aggression—for instance, being fired upon, shooting at the enemy, and exposure to dead bodies or human remains—were more strongly correlated with fearlessness about death than more benign experiences, such as disarming civilians, seeing physical devastation, and being in an accident. The results of these studies lent support to the hypothesis that the capability for suicide could develop or be acquired over time as a result of accumulated exposure to painful and provocative experiences. These findings strengthened our confidence in the deployment-suicide link even more.

By that point, we had essentially supported two links in the chain that was assumed to connect deployments with suicide risk: (1) combat exposure was related to fearlessness and pain tolerance; and (2) fearlessness and pain tolerance were related to suicidal thoughts and behaviors. We had not yet, however, connected these two separate links of the chain into a single continuous one—a critical step for testing the theory. If we could not connect these links, we would be unable to claim that deployment was related to suicide *because* it increased fearlessness and pain tolerance.

To illustrate the importance of this extra step, let's take a moment to think about the relationships among three very different things: air conditioner use, seasons of the year, and sunburns. Air conditioner use is positively correlated with the summer months because that's the time of year when temperatures are highest. Summer months are also positively correlated with sunburns because people spend more time outdoors, increasing their exposure to sunlight. Air conditioner use is also correlated with sunburns, but not because air conditioners *cause* sunburns. Rather, the correlation of air conditioner use and sunburns is explained by something else entirely: increased exposure to sunlight, which happens to coincide with summer months, higher temperatures, and people spending more time outdoors. A is therefore correlated with B, B is correlated with C, and A is correlated with C, but this does not necessarily mean that A causes C.

Achieving this objective—connecting the links among combat exposure, fearlessness and pain tolerance, and suicidal thoughts and behaviors—became a primary focus of my research, but despite repeated attempts, we were never successful, no matter how we approached the problem or analyzed the data. We simply could not conclude that combat exposure was related to suicidal thoughts and behaviors because of increased fearlessness and pain tolerance. It was incredibly frustrating. Unable to confirm what I was certain was true, I eventually set this line of research aside.

A Shift in Mindset

In 2010, while I was working on this problem, the Army released a comprehensive report noting that approximately 70% of Soldiers in the Army had previously deployed. The proportion of Soldiers who had died by suicide and had previously deployed was also around 70%—a nearly identical value. This was an unexpected finding for most of us who believed that the rise in military suicides was attributable to increased deployments. If deployment really was causing the increase in military suicides, we would have expected deployments to be more common among those who died by suicide as compared to those who did not. What the data actually suggested was that Soldiers who had died by suicide *were no more or less likely to have deployed than other Soldiers*. This single data point certainly was not definitive and did not completely rule out the possibility that deployments were increasing suicide in some unknown way, but it didn't fit with the hypothesis. It did, however, fit with what I was finding in my own research: no relationship. I started to second-guess my original assumptions about the deployment-suicide link. Perhaps I was wrong. Perhaps increased deployments didn't explain the rise in military suicides after all.

In the years to follow, multiple large-scale studies similarly failed to support a correlation of deployment history with suicidal thoughts and behaviors. In the Millennium Cohort Study, for instance, an enormous study of more than 150,000 military personnel who served during or after 9/11, Cynthia LeardMann and colleagues found that the suicide rate among those who had deployed was not meaningfully different from the suicide rate among those who had never deployed. The year after that, the Army Study to Assess Risk and Resilience in Servicemembers (Army STARRS) concluded that the rise in military suicides from 2004 to 2009 was similar for Soldiers who had previously deployed and Soldiers who had never deployed. Soon thereafter, a third team of military researchers led by Mark Reger analyzed records from all of the 3.9 million military personnel who had served in the U.S. military from 2001 to 2007 and found that suicide rates among those who had deployed and those who had not were nearly identical.

For every one of these studies, there seemed to be another study supporting the opposite conclusion: deployment *was* correlated with suicides. A separate study from the Army STARRS team reported that Soldiers who had deployed two or more times were more than twice as likely to have attempted suicide after joining the military. In two separate studies, Shira Maguen and colleagues found that killing in combat was associated with increased risk for suicidal thoughts in both Vietnam-era veterans and Iraq- and Afghanistan-era veterans. In my own research, combat exposure was correlated with suicidal ideation among active duty Air Force personnel, but only for personnel who were above the age of 29 and reported low levels of belongingness. From 2011 to 2015, it seemed as though each new study that had something to say about the presumed deployment-suicide link just muddied the waters even more rather than clarifying the issue. Based on my own read of these many studies, it seemed clear that the overall weight of evidence leaned much more toward the conclusion that deployment was *not* correlated with suicide risk. Other researchers arrived at the opposite conclusion based on their own interpretation of these same studies. Unfortunately, the clear, simple answer that we all desired and sought remained elusive.

Amidst this back-and-forth debate, Peter Linnerooth, a clinical psychologist who had served in the Army and deployed to Iraq, died by suicide. I did not know Pete personally, but the military mental health community is small, such that most of us who served are only a few degrees of separation from just about every other military mental health professional who is currently serving in the military or who served in the recent past. I was only two degrees of separation from Pete, linked to him via a mutual colleague.[3] I was working at my computer in my San Antonio office when the news about Pete's death arrived via e-mail. In his e-mail message, our mutual colleague wrote that although he respected my research and understood why I did not believe that deployment was correlated with suicide, he did not (and could not) agree with that conclusion. Deployment had changed Pete, he explained, and had set into motion the slow downward spiral that led to his death. As I learned more about him, I couldn't help but to arrive at the same conclusion: Iraq had had a profound effect on Pete. Indeed, I found it impossible to conclude that his experiences while deployed had nothing to do with his suicide. Pete's death prompted me to reconsider, yet again, my position on the deployment-suicide correlation. We were very clearly missing something important, but it wasn't clear what it was. I therefore returned to this line of research, albeit with less certainty about how to approach the question or conviction about what the answers would probably be.

This shift in mindset allowed me to consider various ideas and perspectives that I had previously overlooked or even dismissed. Rather than seeking to determine if one answer or idea was "right" (which implicitly assumed the competing answer or idea was "wrong"), I sought instead to understand what might be contributing to these competing perspectives, and (most importantly) allowed for the possibility that there might not be a right or wrong answer at all. This shift in mindset ultimately proved invaluable.

Finding Patterns Amidst Conflicting Evidence

When some studies suggest one conclusion and other studies suggest the opposite conclusion, it's possible that one of these two sets of studies is completely wrong and the other is completely right. Another possibility is that some overlooked factor or explanation is exerting some sort of influence that isn't immediately apparent. I started searching for every published study I could find that had examined how suicidal thoughts and behaviors might be related to deployment among military personnel and veterans, reading each paper and report in detail as I found them. Over the course of a year, I identified 22 studies and reports that addressed the issue. Some of these studies suggested that suicidal thoughts and behaviors were more common or more severe among military personnel and veterans who had deployed, but other studies failed to find this relationship.

Obtaining seemingly contradictory results and arriving at different conclusions is reasonably common in science for a number of reasons. For instance, researchers may use different procedures to collect data, and they may make different decisions about how to analyze those data. Patterns and relationships among variables and factors also can differ across various groups of people and populations; men may respond differently than women, younger people may respond differently than older people, Soldiers may respond differently than Marines, and so on. In this sense, the confusion surrounding the deployment-suicide correlation was not all that unique; similar situations have occurred many times before in all branches of science, not just the psychological sciences. Because of this, researchers have developed methods and strategies to sort it all out. One such strategy is called a *meta-analysis*.

A meta-analysis is sort of a "study of studies" or, perhaps more accurately, an "analysis of analyses." In a typical research study, a researcher collects data from individual participants and then analyzes the data to identify trends or patterns across everyone who participated in the study. For example, we might calculate the mean score for some variable across everyone, or we might calculate the correlation between two variables so we can see how strongly they are related to each other. In a meta-analysis, however, researchers seek to identify trends or patterns across the results of multiple analyses coming from multiple studies. In contrast to the typical research study in which individual *people* provide the data to be analyzed, in a meta-analysis, the individual *studies* provide the data to be analyzed. If done well, a meta-analysis can be a very powerful type of research study because it provides a way to summarize the results and conclusions of many other research studies. One especially useful purpose of a meta-analysis is to potentially identify explanations for why some studies support one conclusion when other studies support a different conclusion. Sometimes, meta-analyses can help researchers to see how, when viewed from a broader perspective, results that appear to differ across many studies do not actually differ so much after all. Like any other scientific method, meta-analyses have limitations that one should consider when interpreting their results, but when conducted rigorously and carefully, they can be very informative.

For my own part, I hoped that a meta-analysis would shed some light on the apparent confusion surrounding the deployment-suicide link. Reading through the 22 papers and reports that I found, one of the very first things I noticed was that different studies used different methods for defining or measuring "deployment." In some studies, researchers simply considered whether or not a service member or veteran had ever deployed and used this yes/no variable in their analyses. In other studies, researchers counted the total number of times that a service member or veteran had deployed, providing a count variable ranging from zero to some upper value. Overall, these two types of studies failed to support the deployment-suicide correlation. In other studies, researchers asked service members and veterans to fill out a checklist that described a variety of events that can occur while deployed. These checklists often included combat-related experiences such as being fired upon, firing one's weapon at the enemy, and seeing dead bodies or human remains. Overall, these studies tended to yield mixed results; some supported a deployment-suicide correlation but others didn't. Interestingly, within this latter group of studies, the deployment-suicide correlation seemed to be consistently supported when researchers focused on one particular type of combat experience—exposure to killing and death—but the correlation was not supported when researchers considered the broader spectrum of deployment- and combat-related events. Researchers also used different indicators of suicide risk—some considered suicidal thoughts, some considered suicide attempts, and others considered suicide death—but these differences didn't seem to impact the results or conclusions very much.

In our meta-analysis, we examined how the results of studies varied across these research methods and schemes. Do we arrive at one conclusion, for instance, if we look at the studies that correlated *deployment history* with suicidal thinking but arrive at a different conclusion if we look at the studies that correlated *killing and death* with suicidal thinking? When we were done with our analyses, our results confirmed that this was the case: Different methods for defining or measuring deployment history and combat exposure made a big difference. Studies that considered deployment history (e.g., *Has someone ever been deployed?*) or total number of deployments (e.g., *How many times has someone been deployed?*) generally found no correlation with suicidal thoughts and behaviors. By contrast, studies that considered exposure to death and killing (e.g., *Has someone been involved in or witnessed someone being killed? Has someone witnessed someone dying?*) consistently found a correlation with increased likelihood of experiencing any suicidal thoughts or behaviors, and a correlation with increased severity of suicidal thoughts. Being deployed, in and of itself, was not necessarily correlated with increased risk for suicidal thoughts and behaviors, but seeing someone die or causing someone's death was. Notably, this correlation seemed to persist even many years after service members and veterans had been deployed.

The deployment-suicide issue highlights several characteristics of wicked problems. First, there is no definitive way to formulate or define a wicked problem. Different researchers, therefore, approached the deployment-suicide question using different methods and strategies. Because there is no one way to define a wicked problem, the problem often is not understood until after the formulation has been developed. The meta-analysis helped to show how different ways of formulating the problem were related to each study's results. Second, solutions to wicked problems are not true-or-false, but some solutions may be better or worse than others. As a result, there is no ultimate, definitive, or "right" way to test a solution to a wicked problem.

None of the methods or strategies used by any of these researchers were right or wrong, although we might reasonably argue that some methods were better suited to the task than others.

Confirmation Bias and Productive Stupidity

When we finally published these findings in 2015, the most common reaction I received was that our results and conclusions were "obvious." Of course, this conclusion was not quite so obvious *before* we had done the analyses. If it had been, there would've been no reason to run the analysis in the first place and there would've been no debate about the matter. This confusion existed because researchers like me were largely focused on determining whether deployment (or combat exposure) increased a service member's risk for suicidal thoughts and behaviors instead of considering *for whom and under what circumstances* might deployment increase this risk. In retrospect, I think people found our study's results to be "obvious" because they tended to interpret the findings in a way that confirmed what they already believed. Those who believed that deployment increased suicide risk zeroed in on our finding that exposure to death and killing was correlated with suicide risk. Conversely, those who believed that deployment did *not* increase suicide risk zeroed in on our finding that deployment history was not correlated with suicide risk. In some ways, it's not surprising that these differences persisted after the meta-analysis was published. Wicked problems are often viewed and understood from multiple perspectives and frames of reference by stakeholders. As noted previously, some of these perspectives may be better or worse than others, but none can really be classified as right or wrong. Even though the results helped to clear up some confusion about the deployment-suicide question, our meta-analysis didn't have much of an impact on people's perspectives and assumptions about the matter at all. This tendency to interpret new information in a way that supports what you already believed is known as *confirmation bias*.

My early research seeking to understand the correlation (or lack thereof) between deployments and suicide among military personnel embodied confirmation bias; I was confident that I knew what was true from the start, and I found evidence to support my perspective. When I ran into contradictory evidence, however, or could not confirm what I believed to be true, I became frustrated and stopped working on the problem instead of considering the possibility that my assumptions were faulty and that I knew much, much less about the matter than I originally thought. The tragedy of Pete Linnerooth's death helped me to accept this uncomfortable truth and to use it to my advantage—to become what is termed *productively stupid*.

I first stumbled upon the idea of productive stupidity by accident several years ago while prepping for an undergraduate class. One of my goals for the class was to foster critical thinking skills and the ability to differentiate between scientifically supported ideas and pseudoscientific ones. As part of my online research for readings, videos, and other materials to use for the class, I came across an essay in the *Journal of Cell Biology*, titled, "The importance of stupidity in scientific research," written by James Schwartz, a professor of microbiology and biomedical engineering. In this essay, Schwartz described how, as a scientist, he often feels stupid but has come to realize that this is how science is supposed to be. Indeed, scientists and researchers find answers to important questions because they are willing to embrace the limits of their knowledge, to be ignorant by choice, and to willingly say, "I don't know." Researchers who become comfortable with this stupidity are willing to consider some of our most important (and in some cases, our most troubling) questions using newer methods or perspectives. These researchers worry less about "failing" or getting things wrong because they realize that being wrong is simply a part of the process. As a result, they are more likely to identify useful answers to important questions because they take more risks and explore new territory. Their stupidity is not a hindrance to their work; on the contrary, their stupidity yields productivity.

Confirmation Bias Within Suicide Prevention

Over the past several years, I have become increasingly concerned that the suicide prevention community has become ensnared in this same bias. When it comes to suicide, we have a tendency to interpret information in a way that supports traditional ideas and concepts, even when the information may not provide much support for these ideas at all or, in some cases, may actually contradict them. Because of confirmation bias, our approach to suicide prevention has remained largely unchanged for years—decades even—despite growing evidence that this approach is not working. Consider, for example, temporal trends for suicide in the United States over the past four decades (see Figure 1.1). From 1986 to 2000, the U.S. suicide rate slowly declined,

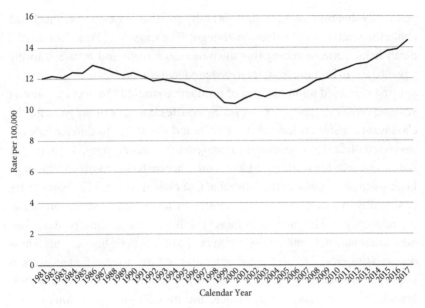

Figure 1.1 U.S. suicide rate, by year, from 1981 to 2017. (Source: National Center for Injury Prevention and Control, Centers for Disease Control and Prevention)

but in 2001 the trend reversed directions and has continued to rise since. According to Centers for Disease Control and Prevention (CDC) data, the U.S. general population suicide rate in 2017 was approximately 33% higher than it was in 2000. In sharp contrast to the United States, suicide rates have decreased since 2000 in approximately three out of every four (to be precise, 137 of 183) nations around the world. Indeed, the U.S. increase in suicides from 2000 to 2016 was the third largest increase in the world (the largest increases occurred in the Ivory Coast and the Republic of Korea). These trends have continued despite an unprecedented rise in public awareness about suicide, a change that has been prompted in large part by a growing number of celebrity suicides in recent years.

In 2014, for instance, Robin Williams died by suicide. In the years immediately preceding his death, Williams had been experiencing a slow and steady decline in cognitive and physical functioning that was initially attributed to Parkinson's disease. In his final months, Williams reportedly experienced severe insomnia, increased confusion, memory problems, mood swings, and intense anxiety. In the months following his death, many in the suicide prevention field worked hard to educate the public about sui-cide. These educational efforts emphasized the message that suicide resulted from untreated or undertreated mental illness, and, by extension, that sui-cide could be prevented by seeking treatment from a mental health profes-sional. More awareness, more screening, and more mental health treatment were needed to prevent tragic deaths like Williams's. As a suicide researcher and clinician, I did my part to support this effort; I fielded questions from journalists, participated in community-based awareness events, and spent extra time responding to questions sent to me via e-mail from individuals who were struggling with suicidal thoughts and family members who had lost loved ones to suicide.

Several months after his death, Williams's autopsy was completed and led to an update in his diagnosis: Lewy body dementia. Lewy bodies are pro-tein deposits that develop in the nerve cells of the brain and are known to cause a range of symptoms including hallucinations, involuntary muscle movements, confusion, memory loss, sleep problems, depression, apathy, and more. Williams's autopsy results suggest that the many symptoms he experienced in the time leading up to his death—the mood swings, the in-somnia, the anxiety, and everything else—probably resulted from Lewy body dementia, rather than from a mental illness such as depression, anxiety, bi-polar disorder, or schizophrenia. Unfortunately, Lewy body dementia has no known cure, and no amount or type of medical or mental health treat-ment could have reversed or offset the progressive nature of this condition. This is not to say that Williams wasn't experiencing depression or anxiety or any other such condition; it's entirely possible to have Lewy body dementia *and* depression. In light of the information available from his autopsy report, however, it seems faulty and potentially misleading to claim or imply that Williams's suicide resulted from an untreated or undertreated mental illness, and that his death might have been prevented by mental health treatment. Yes, Williams was reportedly experiencing symptoms and problems that are often seen in mental illness, but this doesn't mean that these symptoms and problems were necessarily *caused* by a mental illness. Coughing and sneezing are symptoms of the flu, but coughing and sneezing do not always mean you have the flu; these symptoms also may be caused by the common cold, sea-sonal allergies, cleaning a dusty room, or smelling spicy food, to name just a few potential causes.

The inherently complex nature of suicide, like any other wicked problem, renders it beyond the reach of causal explanations such as mental illness.

Nonetheless, many in the suicide prevention community fell victim to confirmation bias, interpreting these symptoms and problems in a manner consistent with what they already believed: Suicide is caused by or results from mental illness. Based on this conclusion, the message was also communicated that mental health treatment can prevent suicide, implying (and in some cases even explicitly stating) that Williams's death could have been averted by mental health treatments—a conclusion that cannot be definitively ruled out as false, even if highly improbable. Unfortunately, the message rapidly spread and took hold, and it lingers to this day.

A few years after Williams's death, suicide prevention catapulted to the forefront of public consciousness again following the suicide deaths of several more celebrities including Aaron Hernandez, Chris Cornell, Chester Bennington, Kate Spade, and Anthony Bourdain. In 2017, the recording artist Logic released a song entitled *1-800-273-8255*—the phone number for the National Suicide Prevention Lifeline—and performed the song live during the 2017 MTV Video Music Awards and the 2018 Grammy Awards— in both cases flanked by individuals who had experienced suicidal thoughts, survived a suicide attempt, or lost a loved one to suicide. Not long thereafter, CNN hosted a town hall on suicide prevention. Seemingly overnight, certain catchphrases that had long been familiar within the suicide prevention community were being repeated over and over again in newspapers, opinion-editorials, television interviews, radio talk shows, blogs, and online memes: *Ask the question, save a life*; *All suicides are preventable*; *Know the warning signs*; *Have the courage to ask for help*; *Suicide prevention is everyone's business*. These catchphrases and messages were not new—they were the same ones recited by suicide prevention advocates for years. It's just that now people outside of the suicide prevention community were reciting them as well. As public awareness of suicide strengthened, the suicide prevention community amplified its calls for more awareness, more screening, more treatment, and more crisis lines—the very same ideas and suggestions that had been recommended for years despite the fact that things were getting worse, not better, as we did these things more often. If something isn't working, doing more of that same thing probably won't work either.

In the midst of this apparent paradox, I found myself second-guessing the status quo, similar to how I felt after Pete Linnerooth's death. On the one hand, I was encouraged by the fact that the general public was now interested in an issue that was so near to my heart. On the other hand, I couldn't help but feel that we were rehashing the same old ideas and promulgating the same old methods despite little (if any) incremental gains or evidence of benefit. I also found myself questioning many of our core assumptions about suicide. How do we know that asking someone if they're thinking about suicide will save their life? How do we know that all suicides are preventable? How do we know what constitutes a suicide warning sign and what does not? How do we know that suicide is caused by mental illness? How do we know that mental health treatment will prevent suicide? If we're so certain about what causes suicide and what needs to be done to prevent it, why are we so *bad* at this? What if we're wrong?

Becoming Productively Stupid About Suicide

When it comes to suicide, we've become stuck, returning to the same old ideas that don't really seem to work, but somehow finding some way of interpreting this failure as evidence of our success. Why? First, our approach to suicide prevention assumes that suicide can be "solved" in the same ways that conventional problems can, for which one or more "correct" solutions exist that can be identified using systematic methods such as trial and error. If a proposed solution to one of these conventional problems doesn't work, we can simply try a different solution instead, repeating this process over and over again until a solution works, thereby fixing or eliminating the problem. Suicide isn't a conventional problem, though; it's a complex and wicked problem with no "right" way to define or conceptualize the problem, and no "right" solutions.

A second problem is that we are generally uncomfortable with this reality because it highlights all that we do *not* know about suicide. We do not know why some people die by suicide and why others do not, and we know almost nothing about why suicidal behaviors occur when they do (e.g., why Saturday evening instead of Saturday morning or Friday afternoon?). Nonetheless, we *believe* that we know certain things about suicide and act accordingly. We fall back on "tried-and-true" ideas and solutions that seem to confirm our beliefs, even though they very clearly have not worked. The suicide rate in the United States is increasing, not decreasing, but we double down on the same ideas and solutions anyway, over and over again. We have fallen victim to confirmation bias, repeatedly finding ways to confirm ideas and assumptions that may not be as accurate or useful as we think. We are uncomfortable with being wrong, so we use well-worn methods that yield relatively small (if any) incremental gains in knowledge because they return results that largely serve to confirm what we already know. This approach feels good because it helps us to feel right, but little of value is ultimately gained.

Getting Unstuck

Productive stupidity, by comparison, benefits more than just the researcher; it also benefits humanity at large. If we want to be better at preventing suicide, we need to become productively stupid. Suicide is a complex, wicked problem that cannot be easily defined and cannot be "solved" or completely eliminated using approaches that work for conventional problems. Some strategies and solutions will work better than others for reducing suicide, but no single solution or combination of solutions can be considered "right" or "correct" because these strategies may only be better than others under certain conditions or circumstances. Likewise, some strategies and solutions will be worse, but cannot be completely ruled out as "wrong," even if they always do worse than other strategies. If we want to be better at preventing suicide, we must adopt a different mindset wherein we become comfortable with these complexities and approach suicide as a wicked rather than a conventional problem.

2

The 90% Statistic

When I was deployed to Iraq in 2009, I carried a sidearm at all times; it's a requirement of all military officers, even noncombatant officers such as I was, who are deployed to a combat zone. Because of this requirement, the first task I accomplished upon arriving in Iraq was to check out a government-issued sidearm, a Beretta M9 semiautomatic pistol, from the armory. The M9 is a short recoil, single-action/double-action pistol that uses a 15-round magazine and serves as the standard sidearm of the U.S. military. Instead of a sidearm, enlisted personnel are issued an M16, a 5.56mm automatic rifle with a 30-round magazine. The M16 was first deployed for widespread military use during the Vietnam War, and is a variant of the AR-15 rifle that has acquired a certain degree of infamy in the United States due to its use in multiple mass shootings. By the time of my deployment to Iraq in 2009, however, a shorter and lighter version of the M16, the M4 carbine, was instead being regularly issued to infantry and other personnel engaged in direct combat.

When I was issued my M9, I also received an olive green government-issued holster attached to a wide green belt that looked like it had been designed (and used) during the Second World War. "No one uses those things," the psychologist I was replacing explained to me, referring to the holster. "They're really uncomfortable and not particularly convenient." He therefore loaned me his leather shoulder holster and said I could use it until I got my own. Later that day, he walked me to the on-base bazaar, which was populated by local merchants selling a range of goods and trinkets including rugs, hookahs, shirts, dresses, and DVDs. The bazaar also had a leather shop that sold a wide range of shoulder holsters—the preferred method for carrying a sidearm. I browsed through the many designs that varied by size, color, handedness, and artwork, and after trying on several, ultimately picked one that I liked. Because I'm right-handed, the sidearm was holstered on my left side, tucked between my left arm and upper torso, somewhat above my elbow. On my right side, tucked between my right arm and upper torso, were two magazines with 15 rounds each.

Although I had handled firearms before and had gone shooting with friends prior to joining the military, this was the first time that I had ever carried a firearm on my person on a regular basis. Because carrying a sidearm was a new experience for me, I initially found the holster to be annoying, mostly because the firearm was constantly banging against my side and getting in the way while I was doing just about everything. When in my clinic, I would therefore remove the holster and place the sidearm in a desk drawer. I only did this a few times, though, because I was prone to leaving the sidearm behind when leaving the clinic, going to the bathroom, or stepping away from the office for a few minutes. This was a grievous error because you're not supposed to leave your firearm unattended or unsecured, so I decided it would be best to just wear the holstered sidearm all the time. Wearing it all the time, I quickly got used to it and it became a part of me. It wasn't until six months later, when I turned the sidearm back in as I was training my replacement and preparing to head back home that I realized just how used to it I had become. For the next few days I found myself constantly distracted by its absence. I felt that a part of me was missing, and I felt naked without it.

The omnipresence of weapons in the day-to-day life of a combat zone also took some getting used to. When you went to the dining facility to eat a meal, there were armed guards standing outside the entrance checking IDs. Inside, dozens or even hundreds of service members were eating together at tables, weapons slung over their backs, resting on the floor at their feet, or holstered at their sides or on their legs. When you went to the gym to work out, people were lifting weights with their rifles resting next to them on the floor or against the wall, always within reach. For my part, I continued to wear my holstered sidearm while lifting weights, or hung it off the edge of the treadmill while running. Just as I got used to wearing a sidearm all the time, I eventually got used to seeing firearms everywhere as well, to the point that they were no more noteworthy than any other common accessory, such as a wristwatch or a pair of sunglasses. Granted, firearms are quite different from these other accessories because of their unique capacity to be deadly, but with enough time and exposure, you sort of forget about that detail as well.

The firearms we carried weren't just potentially deadly for our enemies— the intended target—they were potentially deadly for us as well. Because of this, we carried our firearms in particular ways and followed certain rules for handling them, all of which were intended to prevent accidental injury. There were no rules or methods for preventing deliberate, self-inflicted injury, though. This reality rarely popped into our conscious awareness, but when it did, it was because someone had died by self-inflicted gunshot wound or had attempted to do so. I remember, for instance, one young Marine, only 19 or 20 years old, who was flown to our hospital after attempting suicide with his M16. Although the decision to send him back to the United States due to elevated suicide risk had already been made by the time I met with him, I was nonetheless called to conduct a suicide risk assessment and address any immediate psychological needs he might have while awaiting the next medical transport home.

An Unexpected Case

When I met with this Marine in the emergency department, his desert-colored digital camouflage utility uniform was still dusty, his hair was matted with sweat, and he had a few days' worth of stubble along his jawline and cheeks. In the midst of this stubble, just off the center line of his chin, was a dark black smear surrounding a laceration approximately one inch long. The black smear was gunpowder residue that had been released from the barrel of the M16 that he had placed under his chin, and the laceration was the consequence of the bullet that had discharged when he pulled the trigger. For whatever reason, despite placing the rifle squarely under his chin, the bullet missed its mark when this Marine pulled the trigger, leaving the small laceration as the sole tissue damage or physical injury.

After introducing myself, I pointed at his chin and asked him if he would be willing to tell me the story of that injury. The Marine described an ordinary day by most combat zone standards: He woke up and prepared for the day's mission, which involved a routine patrol in armored vehicles through the city. The weather that day was also typical by most summer-in-Iraq standards: sunny and hot, with the high temperature exceeding 110 degrees Fahrenheit (43 degrees Celsius). After several hours of an uneventful patrol, his convoy started its return trip to base. At some point during this hour-long leg of the journey, the Marine reported that he "saw this image in my mind of me shooting myself, and I just couldn't stop thinking about it." He attempted to push the image out of his mind and to think of other things, but was unable to do so for the remaining 30 to 60 minutes of the patrol. When the convoy finally returned to base, they headed to the motor pool to park, at which point the Marine hopped off the vehicle, placed the rifle under his chin, and pulled the trigger.

I've spent a lot of time in the years since wondering about how that Marine "missed." One possibility I've considered is that the suddenness of the act caused him to pull the trigger before it was firmly seated under his chin. Another possibility is that he lost his grip, allowing the muzzle to shift far enough forward that the bullet only grazed the front of his chin. Yet another possibility I've considered is that some part of him still wanted to live and jumped into action, moving his hands or his head just enough to survive. Maybe it was some combination of these possibilities, or maybe there is another explanation entirely. I'll never know for sure, but what I do know is that right after that Marine pulled the trigger, he was tackled almost immediately by his peers, his weapon was secured, and he was transported to our hospital, where I was able to talk with him and listen to his story.

The results of my evaluation indicated this Marine had no prior history of suicidal thoughts or behaviors and no prior history of mental illness or mental health treatment. The first time he had ever experienced suicide-related thoughts or imagery was on that day, less than an hour before he made the suicide attempt and only a few hours before I met him. He hadn't been drinking alcohol or using any other substances or narcotics at the time—the toxicology lab results confirmed this—and he wasn't having any particular problems with his sleep in the preceding weeks. He wasn't experiencing symptoms of depression or traumatic stress, he wasn't expressing any hopelessness or negative thoughts about himself, and he wasn't experiencing any significant problems in life; no marital or relationship conflict, no financial hardship, and no pending or recent disciplinary actions. When I asked the Marine about his day, he described a routine, benign day. Nothing bad or out of the ordinary had happened, and he hadn't been feeling especially stressed out. He had no discernible risk factors for suicide other than being a young, White male. I checked in with his supervisor and commander, who had come to the hospital with him, and they confirmed, to the best of their ability, all of the information he had provided. The case was utterly bewildering; it just didn't make any sense to me. It didn't make any sense to the Marine, either. "I don't know why I did it," he explained, shrugging his shoulders. "It just happened."

How could someone with such a clean bill of health come so close to killing themselves? If I'm completely honest, the Marine pretty much scared the hell out of me. I agreed that he should be medically evacuated out of Iraq as soon as possible, and I filled out the remaining paperwork to do so. A few days later, I participated in a weekly conference call hosted by the Department of

Behavioral Health at Landstuhl Regional Medical Center in Germany—the first stop for medical casualties leaving Iraq. These weekly conference calls included representatives from all of the behavioral health teams scattered across Iraq and were designed to facilitate the transfer of care for service members who were evacuated for psychological or behavioral reasons. When it was time for me to discuss this Marine, I shared what I had learned about him as well as my hope that the Landstuhl team might be able to provide the missing pieces of the puzzle. I was dismayed to learn that after multiple days of observation on an inpatient unit, repeated interviews and assessments by psychiatrists, psychologists, and social workers, and multiple discussions with the Marine's chain of command, they were just as stumped as I was. I was hoping that my colleagues could unlock this mystery for me, and they were hoping that I might have some information or insight that could do the same for them. The case seemed to defy everything we understood about suicide.

The 90% Statistic

Up until meeting that Marine, I fervently believed that suicide was caused by mental illness and could be prevented by treating or reducing mental illness and its associated symptoms and problems. I also believed that all suicides could be prevented; it was just a matter of recognizing warning signs and intervening early. I certainly didn't come up with these ideas on my own; they were (and continue to be) central axioms of the suicide prevention community and society more generally, and I had never really questioned them or wondered about the information upon which they were based. Like most who are actively involved in suicide prevention, I had learned that 90% of those who die by suicide were struggling with a mental illness at the time of their death. I was also aware that many suicide prevention advocates, including several prominent suicide researchers, believed that 90% was an underestimate—the true value was probably 100%. In other words, *everyone* who dies by suicide has a mental illness. This single statistic certainly is not the only contributor to the perspective that suicide is the consequence or outcome of mental illness—what I will call the mental illness model of suicide—but I would argue that this statistic serves as its keystone.

The 90% statistic comes from a 2003 study conducted by a team of researchers led by Jonathan Cavanagh. In that study, Cavanagh's team compiled the results of 76 separate studies using a research method called the *psychological autopsy*. The psychological autopsy involves collecting and reviewing as much information about the decedent as possible from sources including medical records, social media accounts, and interviews with family members, friends, and healthcare providers. As a method, the psychological autopsy was originally developed to clarify the mode of death in cases where it was unclear how an individual died. For example, did a decedent kill herself or was she murdered by an angry ex-husband? Did a decedent accidentally overdose on his medication, suggesting an accidental death, or did he deliberately overdose, suggesting suicide? When conducting a psychological autopsy, the individual conducting the review typically examines the factors surrounding the individual's death, information known about the decedent, and observations made by others who knew the decedent, such as family members, friends, and coworkers. If these various sources of information suggest the decedent was experiencing a psychological disorder (e.g., medical records might show they were in therapy and/or taking psychiatric medications, or family members might report observing social withdrawal and verbalizations about suicidal intent), the probability of the death being a suicide is assumed to be higher. If, on the other hand, the decedent was not actively engaged in mental health treatment, was performing well at work, and was socially active and engaged with family and friends, suicide may be deemed less probable.

Although the psychological autopsy was initially developed to help clarify questions regarding a decedent's manner of death, it was eventually adopted by researchers as a tool for understanding risk and protective factors for suicide. One leading risk factor of interest to researchers is the presence (or absence) of mental illness. Unfortunately, because the majority of individuals who die by suicide did not pursue mental health treatment prior to their deaths, there isn't always any clear or direct evidence to support the diagnosis of a mental illness. Researchers therefore attempt to infer this possibility from the observations and reports of other people who knew the decedent. Did they appear sad? Were they less energetic than usual? Were they restless and on edge? And so on. Researchers then make their best guess based on this information.

Across 76 psychological autopsy studies, Cavanaugh's team found that the median percentage of suicide cases who were retrospectively (i.e., after the individual had died) diagnosed with a mental illness was 90%. This rule didn't seem to apply to that Marine, though. For many years, I assumed that he was simply one of the estimated 10% of people who don't have a mental illness when they attempt suicide. At the time, however, in the absence of any evidence to support the presence of a mental illness, I diagnosed the Marine with an adjustment disorder, a diagnosis that refers to the development of "clinically significant" emotional or behavioral symptoms in response to an identifiable stressor. I wasn't able to identify any stressor and neither was the Marine, but my assumption was that a stressor *must* have occurred, otherwise he wouldn't have made a suicide attempt. The Marine also wasn't describing any emotional symptoms of significance, but I reasoned that a suicide attempt certainly met the criteria for a "clinically significant" behavioral symptom, thereby justifying a diagnosis of adjustment disorder.

Over the years, I've talked about this case with colleagues to get their input and perspective. The most common suggestion is that the Marine had a mental illness of some sort that was missed because he was actively concealing his symptoms or withholding information from me. If not, then his symptoms and mental illness must have been disguised in some other way. Perhaps he had experienced a psychotic episode, for instance, or maybe his behavior was the manifestation of an underlying personality disorder, which can be difficult to diagnose reliably during a first appointment or meeting. The Marine was certainly in the right age range for a first psychotic episode—psychotic episodes typically first emerge in early adulthood—but there was no evidence that he was experiencing, or had experienced, any hallucinations or delusions. Aside from my own meeting with this Marine, the behavioral health team at Landstuhl had considered these possibilities as well and ruled them out after observing him for several days and conducting multiple tests and assessments designed to detect these possibilities. The behavioral health team also didn't see any indicators of a personality disorder or any other mental illness, for that matter.

Despite the absence of evidence supporting the presence of a mental illness, the general consensus of the mental health professionals who learn about the case continues to be that there must have been *some* kind of mental illness. Nearly lethal suicidal behaviors don't just happen out of the blue, of course, and we all know that 90%—maybe 100%—of suicidal behaviors are associated with a mental illness. Based on this logic, the conclusion was that the probability of the Marine *not* having a mental illness was low. Just about every mental health professional with whom I have shared this story has agreed that, under the conditions within which I met the Marine (i.e., no evidence to support a mental illness diagnosis), a diagnosis of adjustment disorder was appropriate for the same rationale I had used in Iraq: *Something must have happened to precipitate the suicide attempt, even if that something was unknown,* and the suicide attempt absolutely met the threshold for a clinically significant behavioral symptom.

Curiously, the accumulated consensus of these mental health professionals actually served to decrease rather than increase my confidence in the conclusion that the Marine had a mental illness. I think this is partly because of the confidence with which these mental health professionals asserted their conclusion, despite the absence of any evidence to support it: It *must* be true that the Marine had a mental illness even if there is no evidence to support it. High confidence despite low evidence is not a good combination, and in some circumstances can be a recipe for disaster. If a particular conclusion lacks supporting evidence, our confidence in that conclusion should *decrease* rather than increase. The conclusion may still be correct, but we should be skeptical rather than certain about its accuracy.

The 90% Statistic Is Probably Wrong

That Marine wasn't the only case I encountered while deployed that seemed to defy the mental illness model. There was also an Airman whose suicide attempt by firearm was interrupted by a coworker who just happened to be in the right place at the right time to intervene. The Airman had been notified that he was receiving an Article 15—a severe form of punishment in the military—and had called his girlfriend in the United States to talk with her about his anxiety and fear about the process. This was the second Article 15 the Airman would be receiving during his short career, so he was in an especially bad situation. His girlfriend didn't respond as he had hoped, though; she expressed frustration that he had "screwed up again" and told him that she "couldn't do this anymore" before hanging up. The Airman tried to call her back but she wouldn't answer the phone. "I just don't know what I'm going to do," he later told me. After my meeting with him, I transcribed his words in a journal as best as I could remember them:

I was in my room yesterday and I was just thinking to myself, "What's the point? I just fuck everything up." So I took out my gun from my holster and loaded it, and held it to my head. I started to pull the trigger, but then my friend came to my door and knocked. She saw me with the gun and asked what I was doing, and I told her. She took my gun away and went and told the Shirt,[1] *and they took me to mental health. If my friend hadn't come right then I'm pretty certain I'd be dead. It just happened so fast.*

Similar to the Marine, this Airman had no prior history of suicidal thoughts or behaviors, no history of mental illness or mental health diagnoses, and no history of substance use. Unlike the Marine, however, there were two clear precipitating events: disciplinary action and rejection by his significant other. Because of the disciplinary action, he had been experiencing increased stress and sleep disruption during the preceding week because he was worrying so much about what would happen to him. These symptoms and problems were well within the range of what would be expected under the circumstances, however; they certainly did not rise to the level of a mental illness. This Airman was also blaming himself for his current situation and was worrying about anticipated negative outcomes, but here again, these "symptoms" were understandable and appropriate to the situation, and they were not interfering with his work or relationships with others. If he had met with me under any other circumstances, I would not have considered his symptoms or reactions to be out of the ordinary, and would not have diagnosed him with a mental illness, not even an adjustment disorder. I would have instead considered these reactions to signal a natural stress response. Nonetheless, I diagnosed this Airman with an adjustment disorder because the Airman did not meet the requirements for any other diagnosis or condition, and I considered the act of holding a gun to his head to meet the threshold for a clinically significant behavioral symptom.

These situations didn't just happen while I was deployed to Iraq; I encountered them outside the military as well. While living in Utah, for instance, I learned that around one third of suicides that were precipitated by an argument occurred *during* the argument and involved a firearm. "It just happened," a patient once told me when I asked him to share the story of his own close brush with death under very similar circumstances. He and his wife were having a heated argument, he explained, and "I just wanted it to stop," so he grabbed his loaded handgun and held it to his head. Thankfully, he stopped himself before pulling the trigger. When I asked him what "it" was that he wanted to stop, he described intense emotional distress: "I just felt completely overwhelmed in that moment." This patient acknowledged that he and his wife had been experiencing strain in their relationship at that time, but he did not describe any symptoms or problems suggesting he was experiencing a mental illness prior to their argument. Sure, he described feeling emotionally overwhelmed during the argument, but feeling overwhelmed during arguments does not constitute a mental illness.

Over and over again, I found myself encountering cases like these, in which a sudden decision was made within the context of a stressful situation. Over and over again, some version of the refrain, "it just happened," was offered as an explanation—in many cases accompanied by a confused shrug of the shoulders and resigned shake of the head. Over and over again, I've been struck by how many of these cases did not involve a history of mental illness or mental health treatment, no known or reported history of suicidal thoughts and behaviors, and little to no evidence of a current mental illness. The prototypical story involved an acute reaction to a life stressor, although sometimes no stressor could be identified at all, but the time course and nature of their reactions did not rise to the level of a mental illness. Indeed, if these people had not engaged in suicidal behavior, their reactions would typically be considered "normal" by most standards and would not have reasonably led to the diagnosis of a mental illness, not even an adjustment disorder.

I want to pause here for just a moment to clarify that I am not attempting to characterize suicidal behavior as normal (or abnormal). Rather, I am emphasizing the point that experiencing intense emotional distress is a normal and understandable human experience, especially when it occurs in response to stressful and/or unpleasant circumstances. Feeling overwhelmed during a heated argument with a loved one is something that many of us have experienced—or will experience—at least once in life, and does not necessarily constitute a mental illness. Feeling despondent and humiliated when we receive a Dear John letter also does not constitute a mental illness; neither does feeling panicked or desperate when confronted with an unexpected and large expense. These types of experiences and reactions are completely natural, even if extremely uncomfortable.

I did not recognize this tendency to label natural human experiences as mental health conditions or adjustment disorders right away. I don't know that there was any particular "Aha!" moment; I just know that over the course of time, I started hearing more and more stories about individuals who had died by suicide but did not seem to have a mental illness or a precipitating stressor. Usually, these stories were relayed to me by family members who were desperate to find an explanation for the sudden loss of a loved one. Many of them were familiar with the 90% statistic and had searched for evidence of a hidden mental illness, but in many instances they could find no evidence to support this possibility. Sometimes it was obvious to me that the family member was overlooking or disregarding obvious (at least to me as a clinical psychologist) signs of a mental illness. In these cases, I offered my thoughts and observations as an alternate perspective that could be helpful to the bereaved. In other cases, however, I was left scratching my head as well, just as bewildered as I had been after I had met with that Marine in Iraq.

For a long while, I reasoned that these cases simply reflected "missing data"; the evidence we were looking for existed *somewhere*, but we didn't know where to look. Absence of evidence is not the same as evidence of absence, though. As time passed, however, several lines of evidence prompted me to think about the issue in a different way, and to recognize that I had fallen into the trap of confirmatory bias, which was leading me to maintain a high level of confidence in a predetermined conclusion despite the absence of evidence to justify or support that conclusion with high certainty.

Epidemiological data do not support the 90% statistic

The first line of evidence came from U.S. national suicide statistics released each year by the Centers for Disease Control and Prevention (CDC). These data are publicly available online from the Web-based Injury Statistics Query and Reporting System, or WISQARS (pronounced "whiskers") for short, and from the National Violent Death Reporting System. If you are so inclined, you can access these data sets yourself and produce a wide array of reports. According to these data, only 46% of U.S. citizens who died by suicide between 1999 and 2016 had a known mental health diagnosis at the time of death, a rate that is nearly half the 90% statistic so often cited (see Figure 2.1). That's a pretty sizable difference. What might account for this?

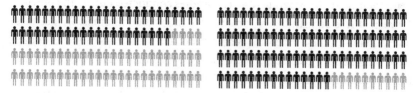

Figure 2.1 The estimated percentage of suicide decedents who have a mental illness at the time of death according to Centers for Disease Control and Prevention data (left) and the suicide prevention community (right).

One possibility is that the CDC's data severely underestimate the prevalence of mental illness among U.S. suicide decedents. In my experience, this appears to be the majority opinion of the suicide prevention community, although a growing number of voices have started to question this assumption. To support this perspective, many have correctly noted that the CDC data only report the occurrence of *known* mental illness rather than the occurrence of *actual* mental illness. Because suicide decedents without a known mental illness are less likely to access mental health treatment than suicide decedents with a known mental illness, this subgroup had fewer opportunities to have their mental illness identified and diagnosed by a trained mental health professional. This is a reasonable argument that is probably true for a certain percentage of suicide decedents without a known mental illness; if every single suicide decedent in the United States had the opportunity to visit with a mental health professional, I do suspect the percentage of suicide decedents who were diagnosed with a mental illness would increase. It's hard to know how much, but it seems unlikely that the increase would be large enough to close the sizable gap between the 46% rate implicated by CDC data and the 90% often cited by experts.

Research studies suggest mental illness is only weakly correlated with suicide

The second line of evidence comes from a recently published meta-analysis conducted by a team of researchers led by Joe Franklin. As a reminder, a meta-analysis is a sort of "study of studies" in which overall patterns of results across multiple studies can be analyzed. Franklin's meta-analysis was designed to summarize what was known about risk factors for suicidal thoughts and behaviors and what new information had been gained about these risk factors over the course of several decades. To do this, Franklin's team identified 365 separate research studies conducted during the previous 50 years; these 365 studies reported more than 4,000 findings. Across these many, many studies, Franklin's team found that indicators of mental illness were only weakly correlated with suicide and suicide attempts, such that, from a prediction perspective, most risk factors were only slightly better than chance when predicting suicide attempts and death by suicide. Although Franklin's study was not intended to calculate rates of mental illness among individuals who died of suicide or attempted suicide, his results can nonetheless provide useful and valuable information.

Franklin reported many of his results using the odds ratio statistic. An odds ratio provides information about how similar (or different) two rates or proportions are across two groups. The statistic, therefore, could provide information about what we might expect the rate of mental illness among suicide decedents to be as compared to the rate of mental illness among people with mental illness who do not die by suicide; the same logic can be extended to those who have attempted suicide versus those who have not. If we assume that 90% statistic is true, that would mean that the odds of as suicide decedent having a mental illness is 9 to 1 because 90% of suicide decedents have a mental illness and 10% do not. We can then compare these odds to the odds of someone who did not die by suicide having a mental illness.

To estimate this second value, we can use the results of the National Comorbidity Survey Replication (NCS-R), a nationally representative household survey of U.S. adults. The NCS-R was designed to be nationally representative, we can be confident that it provides a pretty good estimate of how common mental illness is among U.S. adults. According to the NCS-R, approximately 25% of U.S. adults meet full diagnostic criteria for at least one mental illness in a typical year, whether depression, anxiety, attention-deficit/hyperactivity disorder, substance use, or something else. This means the odds of an adult having a mental illness is approximately 1 to 3, or 0.33, because 25% of people have a mental illness each year and 75% do not. If we assume that these values apply to those who die in any given year (i.e., 25% of those who die each year have a mental illness), we have everything we need to calculate the expected odds ratio of mental illness among suicide decedents as compared to people who die of other causes. To calculate this odds ratio, we divide the odds of a suicide decedent having a mental illness (9) by the odds of a nonsuicide case having a mental illness (0.33), yielding a value of 27. If the 90% statistic is true, we therefore would expect Franklin's odds ratios estimating the relationship between mental illness and suicide to be somewhere in the ballpark of 27.

None of Franklin's results come anywhere close to this value, though. For externalizing disorders such as substance use disorders, the odds ratio was around 1.5; for internalizing disorders, which include mood and anxiety disorders, the odds ratio was around 1.3; and for mental illness in general, which included the presence of any diagnosis and total number of diagnoses, the odds ratio was around 1.7. Odds ratios were slightly higher for suicide attempts as compared to suicide deaths, but not by much: 2.1 for general mental illness, 1.6 for internalizing disorders, and 1.3 for externalizing disorders. These results suggest that a much smaller percentage of individuals who attempt suicide or die by suicide report or show various indicators of mental illness.

What would the odds ratio be if only 46% of suicide decedents have a mental illness at the time of death—the percentage implicated by the CDC's data? We can use the same series of steps to calculate this. If the CDC's estimate is true, then the odds of a suicide decedent having a mental illness would be 46 to 54, which is equal to 0.85 (because 46 divided by 54 equals 0.85). When we divide 0.85 by 0.33, we get an odds ratio of 2.6. This value is still higher than Franklin's estimates, but not by much, which suggests the CDC data and Franklin's results are more similar to each other than the 90% statistic.

Results of treatment studies suggest mental illness is unrelated to suicidal behaviors

The third line of evidence comes from published clinical trials testing the efficacy of various types of psychological treatments for the prevention of suicidal behaviors. To date, only two psychological treatments have been shown to reduce the incidence of suicidal behaviors in multiple treatment studies: dialectical behavior therapy (DBT) and cognitive behavioral therapy for suicide prevention (CBT-SP). Other psychological treatments, such as the attempted suicide short intervention program and mentalization-based psychotherapy, have reduced the incidence of suicidal behaviors in a single study, but these findings have not yet been replicated, so conclusions regarding their effectiveness remain a bit more tentative. We'll discuss these treatments in greater detail in Chapter 6, but for the purposes of our conversation right now, I'll note that all of these treatments, which we can collectively refer to as "suicide-focused treatments," have a good deal in common with one another. When we look across the many studies that have compared suicide-focused treatments to status quo mental health treatments that are widely used by mental health professionals, an interesting pattern emerges. First, suicide-focused treatments consistently reduce suicide attempts by 50% or more as compared to status quo treatments. Second, reductions in depression, hopelessness, anxiety, and other indicators of emotional distress among individuals who receive suicide-focused treatments are comparable to reductions among individuals who receive status quo treatments. In other words, many different types of mental health treatments reduce depression, but only a handful of treatments have also been shown to reduce the probability of suicidal behaviors. If mental illness *caused* suicidal behavior, we should expect that treatments that reduce depression and/or other symptoms of mental illness would be just as good at reducing suicide attempts, but that's not what we see at all. This pattern suggests that whatever works to reduce the probability of suicidal behaviors in suicide-focused treatments, it's not improvements in depression.

Mental health diagnoses are often unreliable

The fourth line of evidence involves the reliability of diagnosing mental illness. Misdiagnosis is a problem that has plagued the mental health professions for decades. A major contributor to this issue is the tendency for clinicians to make diagnoses based on informal methods and procedures that often use one or more nonsystematic and untested "rules of thumb." Luckily, a number of tools exist to improve the accuracy of diagnosing a mental illness: structured diagnostic interviews and validated symptom checklists, for instance. Unfortunately, few mental health professionals use these tools in their clinical practice. Another issue that impacts the reliability of diagnosis is healthcare insurance policies that often do not pay or reimburse mental health professionals for services provided to a patient who does not have a diagnosis that meet's the company's payment criteria. If, for example, someone visits a therapist because they would like to receive some professional support while going through a breakup with a romantic partner, the therapist may only receive payment by the patient's insurance company if they diagnose a mental illness such as major depressive disorder. This applies to suicidal thoughts and behaviors as well: If someone who attempts suicide is not diagnosed with certain mental health conditions, the mental health professional may not be paid for any treatment provided. Under these circumstances, mental health professionals are incentivized to diagnose someone with a mental illness even if that person doesn't actually meet all of the criteria for a diagnosis or is experiencing a reasonable and otherwise normal stress response. This is where the aforementioned adjustment disorder often comes into play.

Adjustment disorder is not a particularly well-defined condition. Because of this, it is frequently diagnosed by mental health professionals when a patient's symptoms and behaviors are not severe enough to meet criteria for another diagnosis. The validity of adjustment disorder is therefore a source of contention among mental health professionals: Research suggests that approximately half of mental health professionals believe the adjustment disorder diagnosis overpathologizes otherwise normal and appropriate responses to stressful life situations; the other half believe the diagnosis is appropriate even when the symptoms and behaviors reported by the individual are appropriate to the situation. Think about that for a moment: Half of mental health professionals are of the opinion that a natural and reasonable response to a stressful situation constitutes a mental illness. It's no wonder that mental health professionals generally view the adjustment disorder diagnosis to have poor accuracy.

While I was in Iraq, I wasn't aware of the questionable reliability and conflicting perspectives about the adjustment disorder diagnosis. To me, a suicide attempt clearly met the criteria for a clinically significant symptom or behavior because suicidal behavior exceeded what I would consider an "expected" or proportionate response to a stressful situation. I suspect that most mental health professionals share that perspective. Over time, however, as I heard more and more stories from individuals who had survived their suicide attempts and family members affected by suicide loss, I found myself thinking about that Marine and all the other cases I've seen and heard about who were similar to him. It occurred to me that in each of these cases, a diagnosable mental illness did not seem to exist *prior* to the behavior's occurrence. If the individual had *not* made a suicide attempt, their reported symptoms and behaviors would not have met the threshold for diagnosing a mental illness at all. If, for example, that Marine had not placed an M16 under his chin and pulled the trigger, he and I never would have met and he would not have been diagnosed with a mental illness. If that Airman who received an Article 15 had not pulled out his gun and held it to his head, his stress, sleep disturbance, and worry would have been considered "normal" for the situation he was in, and he would not have been diagnosed with a mental illness. If that Soldier hadn't shot himself in the head during the morning briefing, there would have been no reason to suspect or assume that he had a mental illness. In each of these cases, there was little evidence that a mental illness existed *before* the suicidal behavior occurred. Furthermore, the suicidal behavior served as the only source of evidence supporting the presence of a mental illness. This pattern suggests our traditional assumptions about the causal role of mental illness for *all* (or nearly all) suicidal behaviors warrants further consideration.

Before moving any further, I want to take a moment to acknowledge that some individuals who attempt suicide have a preexisting, albeit undiagnosed, mental illness because they never sought treatment. For these individuals, the suicide attempt often brings them into contact with the mental healthcare system for the first time, at which point a previously undiagnosed mental illness is recognized and diagnosed. I'm not arguing that these individuals did not have a mental illness to begin with. Rather, I'm arguing that *some* who attempt suicide or die by suicide, perhaps more than we have traditionally assumed, probably do not have a mental illness at all. This latter group might be experiencing significant emotional distress, and this emotional distress may have pushed them toward suicidal behavior, but emotional distress is not the same thing as mental illness.

I should emphasize again that I am not arguing that suicidal behavior is a "normative" or "expected" behavior or response to a stressful situation; suicidal behaviors are extreme, and they are not typical components of natural stress responses. Relatedly, I want to assert that I absolutely consider suicidal behavior to be a "clinically significant" issue. As I will explain shortly, however, I am instead arguing that one of our key assumptions about suicide—that it is always or almost always caused by mental illness—is questionable because it is based on faulty logic, namely confirmation bias.

Suicide Is Not Always Caused by Mental Illness

After much reflection on these issues, I've come to realize that I diagnosed that Marine in Iraq with an adjustment disorder based in large part on two ideas: (1) 90% or more of individuals who attempt suicide have a mental illness, and (2) suicidal behavior results from mental illness. Because of these two assumptions, it seemed impossible to me that suicidal behavior could possibly occur in the absence of a mental illness. I suspect that if I were to conduct a poll of suicide researchers, mental health professionals, suicide prevention advocates, and members of the general public, the overwhelming majority would agree with that statement. If I then were to ask why they agreed with the statement, I'm confident that they would cite the

90% statistic or say something along the lines of "because suicide is caused by mental illness."

The 90% statistic has become a central axiom of the suicide prevention community, a presumed Truth that underlies the overwhelming majority of contemporary research and prevention efforts. Indeed, the 90% statistic is so ubiquitous that it is frequently cited in scientific studies, displayed on suicide prevention websites, and highlighted as a key talking point for public education and outreach campaigns without any citation or reference to its source. The statistic has become a self-evident fact—a truism—and often is discussed in that way: "It is well-known that over 90% of individuals who die by suicide had a mental illness," for instance, which is akin to saying "It is well-known that the sky is blue" or "It is well-known that the Earth revolves around the Sun." The 90% statistic spread like wildfire across the suicide prevention community, achieving the status of fact within a few short years of being published. There are a lot of good reasons for doubting the accuracy of this "fact," though, owing to its nearly exclusive foundation in the psychological autopsy method, a technique that is highly vulnerable to a number of systematic biases and sources of error. Heidi Hjelemand and colleagues, in particular, have articulated several potential sources of error when using the method to diagnose a mental illness in someone who is dead.

Confirmation Bias Contributes to the 90% Statistic

Psychological autopsies often use assessment and interview procedures that are not standardized and have not been researched to determine whether they are reliable and valid. Different interviewers, therefore, may ask different questions, may interview different types of people, and may collect different types of information. Psychological autopsy studies also do not necessarily take into account the potential biases of the family members, friends, and other people who are interviewed. This is important because an interviewee's assumptions about suicide can bias their answers. A family member, friend, or coworker who believes suicide results from mental illness, for instance, may be more likely to retrospectively interpret information as evidence of a mental illness. Someone who believes suicide to be morally or spiritually objectionable, by contrast, may have a tendency to downplay or minimize information that very clearly suggests a mental illness. The possibility of biased responding is increased even more if the person being interviewed is experiencing grief or a mental illness themselves, both of which are known to increase the tendency to report or describe symptoms of mental illness in others. Bias doesn't just influence the people being interviewed, however; bias also can influence the researcher conducting the interviews. A researcher who believes that suicide results from mental illness may be more likely to ask questions about depression and anxiety, and to interpret certain pieces of information as evidence of a mental illness. All of these issues increase the likelihood of error. To illustrate these issues, let's consider a hypothetical example.

Becky's brother, Jim, died by suicide a few months ago. Becky believes that suicide is the result of mental illness. This belief was reinforced by her grief counselor, who told her that 90% of suicide decedents have a mental illness. The grief counselor also provides Becky with some reading materials from a large suicide prevention organization that highlights the 90% statistic and emphasizes the importance of "getting help" in the form of mental health treatment to prevent suicide. Those same reading materials also list the following warning signs of suicide: thinking about death or suicide, depression, mood swings, anger or irritability, social withdrawal, sleep problems, and anxiety or agitation. Based on these various sources of information, Becky assumes that Jim must have had a mental illness that she did not recognize. "How did I not see it?" she asks herself. Becky starts to think back to all of the conversations, get-togethers, and interactions she had with Jim in the time leading up to his suicide. As she's doing this, Becky recalls a time about a month before Jim's death when she asked him to join her and their mother for lunch, but Jim declined the invitation, saying he was behind at work and was trying to catch up. Becky didn't think much about it at the time, but in retrospect, Becky thinks it's interesting that he declined the invitation because usually he would accept. This memory reminds Becky of a text message conversation she had with Jim a couple days before he died. During the conversation, Jim seemed less talkative than usual and made a comment about unexpected bills he had to pay, so he was taking extra shifts at work. Because he was working double shifts, Jim said he was tired all the time and wasn't getting as much sleep as usual. The final text message he sent on that day said, "I'm just so stressed about all this. I can't wait for it to be over." Becky was supportive and said she wished she could do more to help, but at that time she just chalked it up to Jim being stressed out. Now, in the months following his death by suicide, the grief-stricken Becky perceives all of these instances as signs of depression. Furthermore, when Jim said that he couldn't "wait for it to be over," Becky sees now that this indicates Jim was contemplating suicide.

Becky is subsequently interviewed by a researcher named Dr. Jones, who is using the psychological autopsy method to understand risk factors for suicide. Dr. Jones believes that suicide is the result of mental illness, especially depression; indeed, the relationship of mental illness and suicide is one of the central topics she is researching. Part of her interview, therefore, is designed to determine what diagnosis (or diagnoses) Jim might have had at the time of his death. Dr. Jones asks Becky many questions about Jim, including questions about Jim's mood, energy level, social withdrawal, sleep, and thoughts about death or suicide—all of which are symptoms of depression. Becky reports that in the month prior to Jim's death, he was very stressed because of finances and work, had turned down invitations to join her for lunch, reported being tired but unable to sleep, and sent her a text message right before his death in which he said, "I can't wait for it to be over." Dr. Jones notes all of this and then asks more questions about any other problems or symptoms Jim might have had before he died. The wording of these questions helps Becky to remember other things she hadn't thought of before: Jim took much longer to respond to text messages than usual, and one time at a family event he fell asleep on the couch, which was atypical for him. After the interview is over, Dr. Jones reviews Becky's answers and determines they support a diagnosis of major depressive disorder: Jim had an elevated level of emotional distress, excessive fatigue, sleep disturbance, social withdrawal, and thoughts about death and suicide.

After completing all of her interview and analyzing her data, Dr. Jones finds that 85% of the suicide cases included in her study can be diagnosed with a mental illness. Because the 85% rate of mental illness among suicide cases is pretty close to the well-known 90% rate, she and other researchers consider her results to be reliable. Based on these results, Dr. Jones concludes that unrecognized and untreated mental illness is a risk factor for suicide and recommends widespread screening for depression and other mental illness to better detect this risk factor and offer early intervention to reduce suicide. Dr. Jones also recommends wider implementation of antistigma efforts as a key suicide prevention strategy, given that stigma is assumed to be a barrier for mental health treatment. Jim, for instance, probably didn't talk about his depression with his sister or seek out professional assistance because he was embarrassed and ashamed, and because he viewed mental illness as a sign of weakness.

It's entirely possible that Jim's sister and Dr. Jones are right about Jim: he may have been struggling with depression and may not have known it. Another possibility is that Jim's work-related and financial stress, unavailability for lunch, fatigue, and text messages to Becky reflected a reasonable emotional response to an inherently stressful situation rather than depression or any other mental illness. Do heightened stress, declined social invitations, and fatigue *always* signal depression? No. Most of us (probably all of us) have missed or skipped a social event due to work or other obligations, but that doesn't mean we were socially withdrawing from others. Similarly, most of us feel fatigued and exhausted when working extra hard, but that doesn't mean we have depression. Along these same lines, is it possible to be stressed about work and finances without having clinical depression? Of course. Most of us have stressed about a work deadline or another work-related responsibility, and most of us have worried over an unexpected bill or expense. This type of stress is a common, typical human experience and does not necessarily reflect a mental illness.

Because Becky and Dr. Jones believe that 90% of individuals who die by suicide have a mental illness and believe that suicide is caused by mental illness, they are much more likely to interpret this information in a way that fits with what they already believe. Dr. Jones is also more likely to ask questions that seek to confirm the presence of a mental illness without asking questions that might disconfirm or contradict the presence of one. When Becky thinks about how to answer these questions, she is more likely to remember and report information that supports the assumed presence of a mental illness while ignoring or minimizing information that might contradict this conclusion.

As a tool for diagnosing mental illness among individuals who cannot speak for themselves, the psychological autopsy method is therefore vulnerable to confirmation bias. This potential for bias and error associated with the psychological autopsy method is almost never mentioned by experts, however. I don't believe that this is malicious or deliberate omission by any means. Rather, it's my impression that most individuals within the suicide prevention community aren't even aware of these issues. In his original report, for instance, Cavanaugh reported that the percentage of suicide cases across all 76 studies who were diagnosed with a mental illness ranged from 23% to 100%. This means that at least one of the studies diagnosed only one in four suicide decedents with a mental illness and at least one of the studies diagnosed every single suicide decedent with a mental illness. That's a pretty wide range, to say the least. Interestingly, Cavanaugh found a similarly wide range of diagnosis among *non*-suicide cases in psychological autopsy studies that included case controls. In those studies, the percentage of individuals who did not die by suicide but were diagnosed with a mental illness ranged from 0% to 91%—an even wider range that essentially amounts to somewhere between no one and almost everyone having a mental illness.

In order to limit the potential influence of studies that obtained unusually extreme results, Cavanaugh calculated 95% confidence intervals, a statistical method used to provide information about how certain we can be about a finding.[2] These confidence intervals suggest the overall rate of diagnosed mental illness among suicide decedents falls somewhere between 88% and 95%, with a median of 90%, and the overall rate of diagnosed mental illness among nonsuicide decedents falls somewhere between 14% and 48%, with a median of 26%. The confidence interval for nonsuicide cases is especially noteworthy when compared to the estimated annual prevalence rate of mental illness globally, which ranges from approximately 4% to 26%, with a median of 12%.[3] Because Cavanaugh's meta-analysis included studies from multiple nations all around the world, we would expect the median prevalence rate of mental illness among nonsuicide cases to be closer to 12%. This suggests that rates of diagnosed mental illness in psychological autopsy studies are higher than we would otherwise expect based on epidemiological studies. Specifically, the percentage of nonsuicide cases diagnosed with a mental illness across multiple psychological autopsy studies (26%) is approximately *double* the expected percentage based on global epidemiological data (12%). If this bias extends to suicide cases—and there's no reason to believe that it doesn't—then the actual rate of diagnosed mental illness among suicide decedents would be reduced by about half, from 90% to around 45%, consistent with the CDC's estimate.

I readily admit that this is a relatively crude way to estimate bias associated with the psychological autopsy method. We don't know just how biased (or unbiased) the psychological autopsy method truly is as a diagnostic tool for mental illness, but we do know that the method is highly vulnerable to confirmation bias, and there is some evidence that the method probably overestimates rates of mental illness as compared to studies using alternative research methods. I therefore can't help but see psychological autopsy research as a self-fulfilling prophecy of sorts: Individuals who believe that suicide is caused by mental illness are influenced to look for and/or interpret evidence in a manner that supports this belief. This circular reasoning has a powerful effect on our perspectives of suicide (see Figure 2.2). Because we believe all or nearly all suicidal behaviors are associated with mental illness, we assume that suicidal behavior is a sign or symptom of mental illness. Because we assume that suicidal behavior is a sign or symptom of mental illness, we diagnose individuals who attempt suicide with a mental illness. Because we diagnose individuals who attempt suicide with a mental illness, we later find that all or nearly all suicidal behaviors are associated with mental illness. This loop is not only self-sustaining, it actually may be contributing to the adoption of even more extreme views on the matter, specifically the increasingly popular perspective that the true statistic is actually 95% or even 100%.

None of this is to say that mental illness is completely unrelated to suicide and suicide attempts; for some who attempt suicide and die by suicide, mental illness is a very real and important consideration. Rather, I'm arguing that the mental illness model of suicide, which is arguably *the* central assumption of suicide prevention, reflects conventional problem thinking instead of wicked problem thinking. Wicked problems like suicide do not have a single or even a finite number of causes. On the contrary, wicked problems are influenced by so many different factors that the concept of "cause" no longer holds much meaning. The mental illness model is one of many possible ways

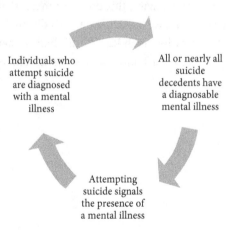

Individuals who attempt suicide are diagnosed with a mental illness

All or nearly all suicide decedents have a diagnosable mental illness

Attempting suicide signals the presence of a mental illness

Figure 2.2 The circular reasoning of mental illness as a cause of suicide. The assumption that mental illness is present in all or almost all instances of suicidal behavior causes us to view suicidal behavior as a sign of illness. Viewing suicidal behavior as sign of mental illness leads us to diagnose individuals who attempt suicide with a mental illness. This reinforces our belief that mental illness is present in all or almost all instances of suicidal behavior.

to think about and understand suicide, but it isn't necessarily the "right" or "correct" way of doing so. The mental illness model may be better than other perspectives of suicide. I would argue, for example, that it is a much better model than one that assumes suicide is caused by demonic possession. This doesn't mean that the mental illness model is better than all other perspectives, however. Indeed, there is considerable evidence suggesting this particular perspective of suicide may not be as useful as we have traditionally assumed, primarily due to its basis in research methods that are highly vulnerable to bias and errors. When carefully considering these multiple lines of evidence, two conclusions are implicated. First, mental illness is only weakly correlated with suicidal behaviors. Second, a much larger percentage of suicides than we may have traditionally recognized occur in the absence of mental illness.

Instead of assuming that most or all individuals who die by suicide have a mental illness, a more balanced and accurate perspective would be that *some* individuals who die by suicide have a mental illness and *some* individuals who die by suicide do not. Likewise, instead of assuming that suicide is caused by or results from mental illness, a more balanced and accurate perspective would be that suicide sometimes occurs within the context of mental illness and sometimes does not. Finally, although mental illness probably influences the emergence of suicidal behavior, this does not mean that it is necessarily *causing* suicidal behavior. As we'll discuss next, traditional ways of thinking about cause and effect may be much less useful than we have long assumed for understanding the conditions under which suicide emerges.

3

Balance Beams and Suicide-Risk Screening

Many years ago when I was working in a primary-care clinic, I met with a middle-aged man whose wife had died by suicide the day before. When he arrived home from work with their two teenage children, they found her body together. The first thing he did the following morning was call our clinic to schedule a walk-in appointment so he could request a prescription for sleep medication and obtain a referral to mental health counseling for his two children. None of the physicians had an available appointment that day, so the nurse asked if he would be willing to meet with me instead, and he agreed. I remember calling for him in the waiting room and leading him down the hallway to my office. As soon as he sat down, he started sobbing. *I don't understand*, he said. *Why did this happen? Why didn't I see this coming? She seemed fine; things didn't seem out of the ordinary. I had no idea she was feeling this way.* In the years since, I've met with many more suicide loss survivors and listened to their stories, whether in a clinical capacity or via e-mail. Their emotions are wide-ranging: some are shocked, some are sad, some are angry, some are embarrassed, some are afraid, some are ashamed, some feel responsible, some are relieved. Many feel more than one of these emotions; some feel them all. In many cases, their questions are the same as the bereaved husband I met with years ago: *What did I miss? What could I have done differently?*

This patient's experience of suicide death as a sudden and surprising event mirrors the experience of many suicide loss survivors that I've met over the years. This isn't always the case, of course; I've also met with suicide loss survivors whose loved one had been struggling for a long time with one or more known mental illnesses, physical illness, and/or persistent problems in life, such as drug use, financial strain, or social isolation. In these cases, their eventual death by suicide was not surprising in the conventional sense of the word, although the specific day and time of the suicide death some-times may not have been expected. Even though these suicide loss survivors are less likely to experience shock and surprise, they nonetheless experience the full range of emotions that accompany grief and loss. For many, however, a loved one's death by suicide is an unexpected event that occurs with little to no apparent forewarning, seemingly out of the blue. The unexpected nature of many suicide deaths stands in sharp contrast to the suicide prevention community's assertion that suicidal behaviors are preceded by warning signs or indicators that signal the behavior's emergence. Recognizing these warning signs, the logic goes, is a critical first step for preventing suicide. Of course, warning signs are useful only to the extent that they can be reliably recognized. Because of this, "raising awareness" about suicide and its warning signs has become a cornerstone of suicide prevention efforts and is a common feature of most public calls to action.

If warning signs exist, though, why are they so often missed? And if we know what signals the emergence of suicidal behaviors, why don't our screening methods and tools work better? In this chapter I will seek to answer these questions. To do so, however, I will present a lot of numbers and use some mathematics, because the whole idea underlying warning signs and screening tools involves probabilities: If a warning sign exists or a suicide-risk screening test is positive, then the probability that suicide will occur soon thereafter is increased. Don't worry, though, I promise that the numbers and math that we use will not be complex or advanced.

Thinking About Suicide or Wanting to Die

Given the dominance of the mental illness model of suicide, it's perhaps unsurprising that public education and awareness efforts have focused on warning signs involving thoughts, emotions, and behaviors. Nine warning signs listed on the websites of several leading suicide prevention organizations in the United States can be found in Box 3.1. These warning signs were derived from the results of studies finding statistically significant correlations of each of these variables with suicidal behavior, studies like those included in Joseph Franklin's meta-analysis and psychological autopsy studies. According to psychological autopsy studies, approximately half of those who die by suicide, on average, express their desire or intent to attempt suicide to others in the time leading up to their deaths, although some studies have found that up to 86% of suicide decedents expressed these desires to others. Psychological autopsy studies also have found that, on average, approximately 16%—one in six—of individuals who die of other, nonsuicide causes also talk about wanting to die or killing themselves prior

---

Box 3.1. Warning Signs of Suicide

---

1. Talking about wanting to die or killing oneself
2. Looking for a way to end one's life
3. Increased alcohol or drug use
4. Withdrawing from others
5. Hopelessness
6. Sleeping too much or too little
7. Feeling anxious or agitated
8. Feeling trapped
9. Anger, rage, or wanting revenge

---

to their deaths. Therefore, talking about wanting to die or killing oneself occurs three times more often among those who die by suicide as compared to those who die of other causes. Given these findings, talking about wanting to die or killing oneself is often prominently featured in public education and awareness efforts. Asking someone if they are having thoughts about death or killing themselves is also a frequently recommended strategy for suicide-risk screening.

Now, you might be wondering at this point about the accuracy of these findings in light of the many problems inherent to the psychological autopsy method that were discussed in the previous chapter. I, too, have wondered about this. For the moment, however, let's set these problems to the side and assume that the statistics are valid: more than half of those who die by suicide—potentially up to 9 out of 10—talk about wanting to die or killing themselves as compared to only 1 out of 6 of those who die by other causes. These statistics would understandably lead us to conclude that talking about wanting to die or killing oneself is pretty common prior to suicidal behavior but not so common other times, and is pretty specific to suicide. If true, why is suicide so often experienced as a surprising or unexpected occurrence?

A critical but often overlooked factor is the imbalance of suicide deaths as compared to all other types of death. In 2017, some 47,173 people died by suicide in the United States and 2,766,330 people died by some other cause (e.g., natural causes, accidents, homicide). Nonsuicide causes of death were therefore 59 times more common than suicide. If the psychological autopsy study results are correct—54% of those who die by suicide versus 16% of those who die by other causes talk about wanting to die or killing themselves prior to their deaths—we can estimate that approximately 25,473 people who died by suicide (54% of the 47,173 suicide decedents) and 442,613 people who died of some other cause (16% of the other 2,766,330 decedents) talked about wanting to die or killing themselves prior to dying. This means that for every person who talked about wanting to die or killing themselves and then died by suicide soon thereafter, there were 17 people who talked about wanting to die or killing themselves who then died soon thereafter of a cause other than suicide. Of note, these numbers include only those who have died. An unknown number of people talked about wanting to die or killing themselves but did not die soon thereafter; they continued to live, resulting in an even larger imbalance. The majority of suicide decedents may therefore show one or more warning signs for suicide but very few individuals who show these warning signs will actually die by suicide.

Let's consider another example. In 2013, Greg Simon and colleagues published the results of a very large research study involving an analysis of electronic health records from a large integrated healthcare system that provided outpatient health services to over 80,000 individuals during a four-year period. In this healthcare system, primary care and mental healthcare professionals administered a nine-item depression symptom scale called the Patient Health Questionnaire-9, or the PHQ-9, at every visit for patients being treated for depression. The PHQ-9 is easily the most widely used screening method for depression and suicide risk in the United States,[1] and its ninth item, which asks patients to report how often they have been bothered by "thoughts that you would be better off dead, or of hurting yourself in some way" during the previous two weeks, is often used as a brief suicide-risk screening tool. Patients can select one of the following four options: *not at all, several days, more than half the days*, or *nearly every day*.

Simon's team was interested in understanding how a patient's response to this ninth item was related to the incidence of suicide death and suicide attempt during the following year. Their results were, in some respects, very supportive of suicide-risk screening: The cumulative risk of suicide attempt and suicide death among patients significantly increased as their self-reported frequency of thoughts about death or self-harm increased. Specifically, patients who reported thoughts about death or self-harm "nearly every day" were approximately 10 times more likely to attempt suicide or die by suicide than patients who reported having these thoughts "not at all." Those are pretty impressive findings. Simon also found that more than half of the patients who died by suicide and around half of the patients who attempted suicide reported some amount of thoughts about death and self-harm on this screening item in the year before they died by suicide. Not surprisingly, these results were quickly picked up by the suicide prevention community and touted as evidence supporting the value of suicide-risk screening. When we translate these results into more practical numbers, however, your enthusiasm may be tempered.

In that study, the risk of a patient dying by suicide within the year after suicide-risk screening was 1 in 3,000 for patients reporting no thoughts of death or self-harm, 3 in 3,000 among patients reporting these thoughts on "several days," 7 in 3,000 among patients reporting these thoughts on "more than half the days," and 10 in 3,000 among patients reporting these thoughts "nearly every day." This means that, for every 3,000 patients who said they were *not* having thoughts of death or self-harm, one died by suicide in the next year and 2,999 did not. By contrast, for every 3,000 patients who said they were having thoughts of death or self-harm "nearly every day," nine died by suicide in the next year and 2,991 did not. The tenfold improvement in identifying patients who die by suicide therefore represented an increase of only eight patients out of 3,000 who were correctly identified, corresponding to an increase in the probability of suicide of 0.03% to 0.3%. In other words, 99.97% of those who said they were having no thoughts of death or self-harm and 99.7% of those who said they were having thoughts of death or self-harm nearly every day were still alive one year later. To me, these numbers tell an important story: Thoughts about suicide or wanting to die should be taken seriously because they reflect being in a vulnerable state, but they do not necessarily lead to suicide.

What if we consider *all* suicide attempts—including nonfatal ones— instead of just focusing on suicide deaths? The numbers are similar, although not dramatically so. For every 3,000 patients who said they were *not* having thoughts of death or self-harm, 12 will attempt suicide in the next year and 2,988 will not, and for every 3,000 patients who say they are having thoughts of death or self-harm nearly every day, 120 will attempt suicide and 2,880 will not. Here, the tenfold improvement in identification is quite a bit better, but we're still left with a discouraging reality: 99.6% of those who say they are having no thoughts of death or self-harm as compared to 96% of those who say they are having these thoughts nearly every day did not make a suicide attempt in the year after they reported having thoughts about death or self. The conclusion here is the same. On the one hand, patients who reported having thoughts about death and self-harm more often were much more likely to attempt suicide or die by suicide soon thereafter, and the majority of patients who attempted suicide or died by suicide reported these thoughts in the preceding year. On the other hand, almost none of the patients who reported thoughts about death or self-harm attempted suicide or died by suicide during the next year. Although these two sentences may appear to contradict each other, both are entirely true.

If you're confused, you're probably experiencing what is known as the *conditional probability fallacy*, sometimes called the *inverse fallacy*. The conditional probability fallacy refers to the tendency to assume that inverse conditional probabilities are equal: the probability of A happening given that B has happened is equal to the probability of B happening given that A has happened. As applied to suicide, the logic proceeds as follows: the probability that someone has reported thoughts about death or self-harm if they have died by suicide is equal to the probability that someone will die by suicide if they have reported thoughts about death or self-harm. If we use the results of Simon's study, we would assume that because 50% to 60% of individuals who attempt or die by suicide previously reported thoughts of death or self-harm, there is a 50% to 60% chance that someone who reports thoughts of death or self-harm will attempt or die by suicide. Unfortunately, this logic is flawed. In reality, 50% to 60% of individuals who attempt or die by suicide previously reported thoughts of death or self-harm but only 0.4% to 4% of those who report thoughts of death or self-harm will attempt or die by suicide in the following year. This imbalance in conditional probabilities results from the very large difference between the number of patients who *think about* death and self-harm and the number of patients who *attempt or die by* suicide (see Figure 3.1). This problem is not limited to suicidal thoughts, of course; all of the purported warning signs of suicide suffer from this same imbalance.

The Dangers of Relying on Warning Signs

What this all reveals is a key challenge for suicide prevention: any given warning sign for suicide will be wrong far more often than it will be right. Even when multiple warning signs are experienced or expressed by an individual, this problem persists. This problem is not unique to suicide prevention by any means; similar challenges exist in other areas of medicine and health. Pressure or tightness in the chest, shoulder pain, and shortness of breath are several well-known warning signs of a heart attack, for instance,

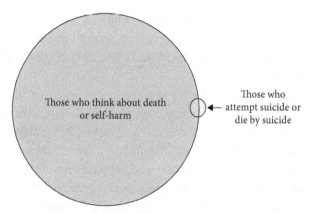

Those who think about death
or self-harm

Those who
attempt suicide or
die by suicide

Figure 3.1 Although more than half of those who attempt suicide or die
by suicide previously reported thoughts about death or self-harm, very few
individuals who experience thoughts of death or self-harm will attempt suicide
or die by suicide.

but these symptoms also are experienced by many people who do *not* have
heart attacks. According to a 2014 study conducted by Holli DeVon and
colleagues, for instance, 63% to 66% of individuals with acute coronary syndrome (an umbrella term that refers to situations in which the blood supply
to the heart is blocked) experienced chest pressure, 27% to 44% experienced
shoulder pain, and 41% to 58% experienced shortness of breath soon before having a heart attack. By comparison, 54%to 64% of individuals *without*
acute coronary syndrome experienced chest pressure, 29% to 34% experienced shoulder pain, and 59% to 61% experienced shortness of breath. The
correlation of these cardiovascular warning signs with an actual heart attack
are therefore small, being similar in size to the correlation of suicide warning
signs and suicide in Franklin's meta-analysis.

If we revisit Franklin's meta-analysis, we can see that individuals with a history of suicidal thoughts at some time during their life are, on average, only
two times more likely to attempt suicide or die by suicide on average than
individuals who have never thought about or attempted suicide. Although a
twofold increase in identifying someone who will attempt or die by suicide
sounds promising, when translated into more easily understood numbers,
our enthusiasm is once again tempered: Approximately 1 in 7,692 individuals die by suicide and 1 in 303 individuals attempt suicide in the United
States each year. If someone reports suicidal thoughts, the likelihood of dying

by suicide in a given year increases to approximately 1 in 6,250, and the likelihood of attempting suicide in a given year increases to 1 in 204. Knowing that someone is thinking about suicide is therefore better than not knowing, but not by much.

Before going any further, I want to pause briefly to clarify that I am *not* arguing against suicide-risk screening; suicide-risk screening is, in my opinion, an important part of comprehensive healthcare delivery. I also want to be clear that these findings should not diminish the importance of responding appropriately to someone who expresses thoughts about death, self-harm, or suicide. Thinking about death and suicide are reliable indicators that things are not going well for someone and that we should render aid or support. If someone says they want to die or want to hurt or kill themselves, we should respond immediately with compassion and concern. My intention in presenting these statistics is to call attention to a very real and important challenge that confronts suicide prevention: poor accuracy and precision in existing screening methods. If we want to do better at preventing suicide, we need to be clear-eyed about the realities that restrict us so we can be productively stupid about how to get around these limitations. What happens if we don't acknowledge these realities? We can become deluded by fallacious thinking and remain stuck.

Disclosure (or not) of suicidal thoughts

One last finding from Simon's study that often is overlooked but warrants some attention is the fact that one in three patients who died by suicide during the study period said they were having no thoughts of death or self-harm when they were last screened, and approximately one in five repeatedly said they were having no thoughts of death or self-harm over the course of numerous medical appointments. Even more alarming is the finding that one out of every four suicide attempts were made by patients who said they were not having any thoughts about death or suicide *less than one week before attempting suicide*. A significant percentage, therefore, of individuals who attempt or die by suicide deny having any suicidal thoughts at all.

Simon is not the only researcher to find this; numerous studies have similarly found that a significant percentage of patients who attempt suicide or die by suicide either deny or do not report suicidal thoughts prior to their deaths. There are at least two factors that contribute to this: (1) individuals may be reluctant or unwilling to disclose their thoughts about death and suicide to others; and (2) thoughts about death and suicide change over time. With respect to the first factor, numerous lines of evidence suggest that non-disclosure and active concealment of suicidal thoughts is common. In one study, for instance, Mike Anestis and Brad Green asked participants in two different ways whether they were having suicidal thoughts. In the first way, Anestis and Green told the participants that their answers would be reviewed by research staff and potentially reported to a military mental health professional so that a full risk assessment could be conducted. In the second way, participants were told that their answers would not be reviewed by or shared with anyone. At the conclusion of the study, Anestis and Green found that one in three participants who reported suicidal thoughts in the second instance (i.e., when their answers were not being reviewed or shared with others) denied suicidal thoughts when they answered in the first instance (i.e., when their answers were being reviewed). Participants were therefore much more likely to disclose suicidal thoughts when they knew that no one would follow up with them about it.

Steven Vannoy and colleagues obtained similar results in a separate study of military personnel. In Vannoy's study, suicidal thoughts were assessed using three different screening tools administered during the same survey. The first tool was a screening survey that military personnel are required to complete after they return from a deployment. Because the screening survey is designed to identify military personnel who may be struggling with a variety of health conditions, including psychological and behavioral conditions, and to connect these personnel with medical professionals, military personnel are required to include their names and other identifying information along with their responses. The second screening tool involved a self-report suicide-risk survey that was not mandated by the military but also asked military personnel to include their names and other identifying information. Finally, the third screening tool was the exact same as the second tool, except it did not require military personnel to include names or any other identifiers at all, thereby preserving their anonymity.[2] When Vannoy compared responses across these three tools, he found markedly different disclosure rates: On the mandated military survey, only 1 out of every 100 participants reported suicidal thoughts; on the identifiable self-report tool, 3 out of every 100 participants reported suicidal thoughts; and on the anonymous self-report tool, 5 out of every 100 participants reported suicidal thoughts. Anonymity therefore increased the willingness of military personnel to disclose thoughts about death and suicide.

Active concealment or nondisclosure of suicidal thinking is not an issue limited to any particular group. In a community-based study conducted by Saskia Merelle, nearly half of the adults who experienced suicidal ideation indicated they had not disclosed these thoughts to others. Merelle's team further determined that nondisclosure of suicidal thoughts was more common among those who reported less severe physical health, less severe emotional distress, and fewer social contacts. Perhaps the most interesting finding from this study is that individuals whose suicidal thoughts occurred infrequently were less likely to disclose their thoughts to others as compared to individuals whose suicidal thoughts occurred more often.

People may be reluctant to share their suicidal thoughts with others for a number of reasons. In an attempt to understand these reasons, Julie Richards conducted a study in which she identified individuals who had attempted suicide less than two months after denying thoughts of death or self-harm on the PHQ-9 administered to them during a medical appointment. Of the 42 patients they identified, 26 agreed to be interviewed. During these interviews, Richards's team asked these patients why they had denied thoughts of death or self-harm when screened by a medical provider. Some patients said they deliberately concealed these thoughts because they were worried that disclosing them would not be helpful, and they expressed fear about how their healthcare professionals would respond. In particular, patients worried that they might be hospitalized. Other patients indicated they were not experiencing thoughts about death or self-harm at the time they were asked to complete the PHQ-9. Still others described having intermittent thoughts about death and suicide that tended to come and go, and felt that the language used to ask about these thoughts did not match their personal experience. To them, the suicide-risk screening item was asking about longer lasting and enduring thoughts rather than fluctuating thoughts.

The ebb and flow of suicidal thinking

This brings us to the second factor limiting the accuracy of suicide-risk screening: thoughts about death and suicide fluctuate over time. The notion that suicide risk ebbs and flows certainly is not a new idea; the dynamic nature of suicide risk is something that has been recognized for at least a century. It's only been within the past few years, however, that this concept has been explicitly researched. Evan Kleiman, for instance, has used a research method known as ecological momentary assessment (EMA) to understand these change processes as they naturally occur in life. EMA involves the repeated assessment of someone's experiences and behaviors in real time as they naturally occur, typically by asking the person to respond to survey items sent via text message or a smart phone app designed specifically for this purpose. In his research, Kleiman used EMA to assess individuals' suicidal thoughts every few hours, thereby obtaining information about how these thoughts naturally change over the course of a typical day. His results indicate that many people experience large shifts in suicidal thinking during time frames as short as a few hours, similar to what's depicted in Figure 3.2. Someone might, for instance, have no suicidal thoughts at breakfast, experience very severe and intense suicidal thoughts at lunch, and then have no suicidal thoughts again at dinner. Variability in suicidal ideation measured over wider time frames (for example, on a daily or weekly basis) also has been observed by other researchers. In my own research, for instance, we found a pattern that was generally similar to that seen in Figure 3.2, although we were assessing suicidal ideation once per week instead of once every few hours.

Traditional suicide-risk screening methods often cannot capture these naturally occurring fluctuations with much precision. If someone experiences large shifts in suicidal thoughts within the span of a few hours, how should they answer a question about thoughts of death or suicide during the past two weeks? Should they indicate how they felt at lunch last week? Should

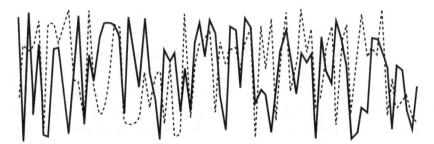

Figure 3.2 Multiple studies indicate suicidal thinking fluctuates over time, sometimes very rapidly and dramatically. This can limit the accuracy and usefulness of suicide risk screening methods, which typically ask about the frequency or intensity of suicidal thoughts during broad windows of time (e.g., during one's entire life or during the past two weeks).

they instead indicate how they felt at breakfast and dinner of that same day? Should they try to average their experiences across these many moments and indicate that as their answer? If so, what if their only suicidal thoughts during the past two weeks occurred during lunch on that one day? How a person responds to questions about their suicidal thoughts also can be influenced by the nature of the question being asked: Does the question ask about the *frequency* of suicidal thoughts or does the question ask about the *intensity* of suicidal thoughts? What if someone was thinking about suicide so intensely during lunch of that one day that he grabbed a firearm, a bottle of pills, or something else that could serve as a method of suicide and started to make a suicide attempt, but then stopped himself just before doing so? What if he hasn't had any suicidal thoughts since that moment? Although the frequency of the suicidal thoughts is low, the intensity is severe enough that he came very close to attempting suicide. Conversely, an individual may have fleeting thoughts about suicide multiple times per day, such that frequency is high but intensity is low.

If thoughts about death and suicide, and warning signs more generally, have such low accuracy and precision as indicators of suicidal behaviors, how can we possibly know when someone is about to attempt suicide? Relatedly, how can we know when someone's alcohol use, withdrawal, and emotional state are indicators of suicide and when they are not? These were some of the questions bouncing around in my head when my wife and primary research collaborator, AnnaBelle, and I moved to Utah in 2012. An unexpected but happy consequence of this move was meeting Jon Butner, a professor of social psychology at the University of Utah who introduced us to *dynamical systems theory*.

Emergence and Dynamical Systems Theory

Dynamical systems theory is a branch of mathematics used to describe the behavior of complex systems. A central focus of the theory is *emergence*, which refers to the process by which a phenomenon comes into existence. Emergence is based on four key assumptions that can be directly applied to suicide (see Box 3.2).

First, change is constant in complex systems. In its most general sense, a system can be defined as a set of things that work together as interacting parts of a network. A system is considered complex when the interactions

---

Box 3.2. Key Assumptions of Emergence

---

1. Change is constant.
2. The whole is greater than the sum of its parts.
3. Each component of a system depends on the other components to function.
4. Complex systems behave in nonproportional ways.

---

among its many components and pieces are so complicated that they cannot be easily understood or modeled. One of the many complications that make complex systems so difficult to understand is their tendency to be in a constant state of flux; systems never really come to rest or settle down. Systems change because they are acted upon by external forces that push them in one particular direction, but these forces are counteracted by built-in regulatory processes that serve to pull systems back to where they started, just as we see in Figure 3.2. If, for example, you are driving on the highway and experience a sudden gust of wind that pushes your car to the right, you are likely to turn the steering wheel left, into the wind, thereby offsetting this external force and reestablishing your position in the center of your lane. We make adjustments like these over and over again while driving in response to ever-changing conditions (e.g., the behavior of other drivers, changes in speed limits, switching from straightaways to curved roadways).

Suicide risk works in a similar way. Under most circumstances, we have a low level of suicide risk. Our suicide risk increases, even if only slightly, when we encounter stressful situations such as relationship problems, financial strain, sleep disturbance, and more; but our suicide risk decreases when we employ strategies designed to offset or counteract these issues. If we feel tired, we may go to bed early. If we are feeling down, we may reach out to a loved one for support or engage in some other activity to feel better. If we are nervous or anxious about a situation in life, we may remind ourselves that "things will be OK" and then mentally work out one or more possible solutions. In combination, we are perpetually being acted upon by the things around us—people, places, and events—and perpetually attempting to counteract or resist the pressure resulting from these external events and situations. Suicide risk is therefore in a constant state of change: periods of increased suicide risk are followed by periods of decreased suicide risk, and vice versa.

The second assumption of emergence is that the whole is greater than the sum of its parts. This refers to the tendency for the combined functioning of a system's many interacting components to create something that did not previously exist, such that the outcome or consequence of change within a system can be completely unexpected or different from any previously observed behavior. As applied to suicide, this assumption implies that the many variables and factors that are correlated with suicide—risk factors, protective factors, and warning signs—interact with one another in highly complex ways that cannot be readily explained by any of these variables and factors by themselves. Things such as depression, hopelessness, trauma exposure, sleep disturbance, perceived burdensomeness, decision-making style, and all other suicide risk and protective factors that have ever been identified are interrelated and influence one another, but none of these variables, by themselves, comes close to explaining suicide. This is, in essence, the central implication of Franklin's meta-analysis: a lot of things are correlated with suicidal behaviors but none of those things has an especially strong correlation and none of those things is sufficient to explain suicide. An important implication of this assumption is that suicide can result from many different combinations and configurations of these same variables. In other words, there is no single "right" combination of suicide risk and protective factors; many, many, many different combinations of these factors can lead to suicide.

Third, each component of a complex system depends on other components of the system to function; no component or piece can operate in isolation. Depression, for instance, is sustained by sleep disturbance and sleep disturbance, in return, is sustained by depression. Hopelessness and perceived burdensomeness are similarly intertwined with each other, such that one is unlikely to exist without the other. Warning signs such as social withdrawal, hopelessness, and sleep disturbance lead therefore to increased suicide risk but increased suicide risk also leads to the intensification of social withdrawal, hopelessness, and sleep disturbance. Because of this mutual interdependence, feedback loops are common instead of linear cause-and-effect relationships, rendering us unable to say that one thing is causing the other. Suicide warning signs and other indicators of mental illness may emerge therefore because suicidal behavior is also emerging, such that warning signs and suicidal behavior emerge *at the same time* rather than one preceding the other. It's like the proverbial chicken or the egg riddle: chickens come from eggs and eggs come from chickens, each one causing and also resulting from the other. If we assume that suicidal behaviors result from linear cause and effect relationships, we can mistakenly assume that suicide warning signs are always apparent before the occurrence of suicidal behavior when in reality this may not always be the case.

The fourth and final assumption of emergence is that complex systems behave in nonproportional ways. This means that small changes within the system can lead to very large differences in the outcome, whereas large changes within the system can have virtually no effect on the outcome at all. Nonproportionality contributes to the weak correlations among suicide risk factors and suicidal behaviors that were identified in Franklin's meta-analysis. Individuals who experience very large increases in depression and hopelessness from one day to the next may not attempt suicide but individuals who attempt suicide may have experienced little to no change in depression and hopelessness from the day before. When small change sometimes, but not always, leads to big differences and large change sometimes, but not always, leads to small differences, the overall net effect is a small correlation.

If these four principles sound familiar to you, it's probably because they have a lot in common with the characteristics of wicked problems, especially complexity. The four principles of emergence align with another mathematical concept that has recently been applied to suicide: *indeterminism*. Indeterminism refers to the idea that an outcome or event (e.g., suicide) is not caused or determined by any particular combination of factors. The applicability of indeterminism to suicide has been most clearly articulated by Joe Franklin (the same Franklin who authored the suicide risk factor meta-analysis). One of Franklin's most frequently used examples to illustrate the concept of indeterminism is to note that there are an infinite number of solutions to solve the mathematical equation $X + Y = 10$. Several possible solutions include:

- $X = 1$ and $Y = 9$;
- $X = 2$ and $Y = 8$;
- $X = 3$ and $Y = 7$;
- $X = 100$ and $Y = -90$; and
- $X = -4588$ and $Y = 4598$.

All of these combinations of X's and Y's equal 10. As a result, all of these many different solutions are correct, and none of the combinations are more (or less) correct than the other; adding together 8 and 2 is just as correct as adding together 3 and 7. These five possible combinations of X and Y values are only a very tiny percentage of all of the possible combinations of values that could equal 10. In the same way, many different possible combinations of risk factors can lead to suicide, none of which are necessarily any more (or less) correct than another.

Implications for suicide-risk screening

An implication of emergence is that change processes generally occur *within* but not *between* individuals over time. In other words, individuals who attempt or die by suicide do not differ in especially meaningful ways from those who do not engage in these behaviors; people who attempt suicide and die by suicide are much, much more similar to each other than they are different. To illustrate, in Figure 3.3 I have plotted the hypothetical fluctuations in suicidal thinking for two different individuals. Both individuals have periods of lower risk and both individuals have periods of higher risk. If we were to administer a typical suicide-risk screening tool to each individual at two separate points in time designated by the arrows, we would arrive at very

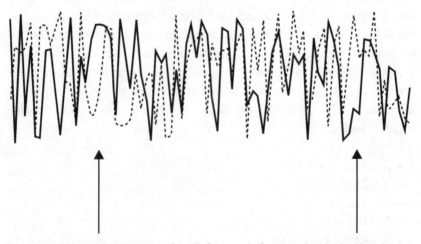

Figure 3.3 Fluctuations in suicide risk for two different individuals who are asked to report their suicidal thoughts as part of suicide risk screening on two different occasions. On the first occasion (left arrow), Person A (solid line) reports severe suicidal thinking and Person B (dotted line) reports mild suicidal thinking. On the second occasion (right arrow), Person A reports mild suicidal thinking and Person B reports severe suicidal thinking.

different conclusions about their likelihood for making a suicide attempt. In the first instance, Person A (represented by the solid line) reports severe suicidal thinking, whereas Person B (represented by the dotted line) reports mild suicidal thinking. We therefore would probably conclude that Person A is "higher risk" than Person B and, by extension, is more likely to attempt or die by suicide. In the second instance, however, the reverse is seen; Person A reports mild suicidal ideation and Person B reports severe suicidal ideation. We would probably conclude that Person B is "higher risk" than Person A and is more likely to attempt or die by suicide. Of course, if we consider the entirety of their timeline, we can see that we would be wrong in both cases and, furthermore, that the two individuals do not meaningfully differ from one another with respect to their overall level of suicide risk. When we compare their scores on a measure of suicidal thoughts (or any other risk or protective factor, for that matter), however, we may mistakenly believe that these two individuals are qualitatively different from each other.

This is because our traditional approach to developing and interpreting suicide-risk screening tools has been largely shaped by approaches designed to distinguish *between* different groups of people, in this case those will who attempt or die by suicide and those who will not. This approach is called signal detection, and it yields a range of concepts that are familiar to many healthcare professionals and clinicians, such as sensitivity, specificity, and positive (and negative) predictive values. To illustrate these concepts of the signal detection approach, consider Figure 3.4, which depicts a group of 100 individuals. Of these 100 individuals, 20 die by suicide (black dots) and 80 do not (gray dots). This is, of course, an enormous exaggeration of the actual suicide rate. If we wanted to more closely approximate the actual ratio of black dots to gray dots in the United States, we would need a figure with 10,000 gray dots for every one black dot—the very embodiment of the expression "a needle in a haystack." To keep things simple for the sake of our current discussion, however, we'll use 80 gray dots and 20 black dots.

Along the horizontal axis of this figure are the scores provided by a hypothetical suicide-risk screening scale. These scores range from 0, which designates lower suicide risk, to 10, which designates higher suicide risk. As you can see, there is a higher density of suicide cases (black dots) on the right hand side of the figure than the left hand side, reflecting the fact that suicide decedents are more likely to have higher scores on the scale. Despite this tendency for suicide decedents to score higher on the scale, a good number of suicide decedents nonetheless obtain low scores. A good number of nonsuicide

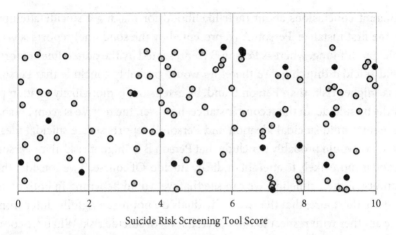

Suicide Risk Screening Tool Score

Figure 3.4 Hypothetical suicide risk screening tool scores for a group of 100 individuals, 20 of whom die by suicide (black dots) and 80 of whom do not (grey dots). In order to identify a larger number of suicide cases, we can set a lower cutoff score. Lowering the scale's cutoff score results in a larger number of positive screens among nonsuicide decedents, however, increasing the false positive rate. Conversely, increasing the scale's cutoff score decreases the false positive rate but reduces the number of suicide cases that are detected. Lower cutoff scores therefore increase sensitivity at the cost of specificity, whereas higher scores increase specificity at the cost of sensitivity.

decedents also score high on the scale, even though we would generally expect them to have lower scores. This mixture of scores across the two groups is a reasonably common pattern for many suicide-risk screening scales.

The purpose of our scale is to identify those who will eventually die by suicide so we can hopefully encourage them to seek out mental health treatment or receive some other intervention. To achieve this goal, we will want to pick a cutoff score that captures the majority of suicide decedents without capturing too many nonsuicide decedents, which are called "false positives." If we have too many false positives, we will have a much harder time knowing who is actually going to die by suicide and who is not, and we may use up limited resources on the wrong people. When we eyeball Figure 3.4, it seems as though a score of 4 might be a good cutoff because most of the suicide decedents scored above this threshold. Using 4 as our cutoff score, we end up with the following results:

- 69 individuals score higher than the cutoff (positive screens) and 31 individuals score lower than the cutoff (negative screens);
- 15 of 20 suicide decedents score higher than the cutoff (true positives) and 5 of 20 score lower than the cutoff (false negatives); and
- 54 of 80 nonsuicide decedents score higher than the cutoff (false positives) and 26 of 80 score lower than the cutoff (true negatives).

These numbers provide us with a sensitivity of 75% (because 15 of 20 suicides, or 75%, are correctly identified as suicide cases), a specificity of 34% (because 26 of 80 nonsuicides, or 34%, are correctly identified as nonsuicide cases), and a false positive rate of 78% (because 54 of 69 positive screens, or 78%, are wrongly identified as suicide cases). Because we have so many false positives as compared to true positives, our scale's accuracy is somewhat low; a positive screen on our scale is correct only 1 out of 4 times.

If we were to increase the cutoff score to 8, we end up with the following results instead:

- 22 individuals score higher than the cutoff (positive screens) and 78 individuals score lower than the cutoff (negative screens);
- 5 of 20 suicide decedents score higher than the cutoff (true positives) and 15 of 20 score lower than the cutoff (false negatives); and
- 17 of 80 nonsuicide decedents score higher than the cutoff (false positives) and 63 of 80 score lower than the cutoff (true negatives).

This provides us with a sensitivity of 25%, a specificity of 79%, and a false positive rate of 77%. Increasing the cutoff score therefore improves the scale's specificity by nearly double but at the cost of sensitivity. We therefore do a better job at identifying those who will not die by suicide but "miss" most of those who will. These changes have little impact on accuracy, however; only 1 out of 4 positive screens continues to be correct.

The key factor that impacts the accuracy of a suicide-risk screening tool (and any medical diagnostic test) is the prevalence of the outcome of interest. In general, the accuracy of screening tools improves when the prevalence of the outcome increases, meaning the outcome occurs more often. In the hypothetical example above, the suicide rate was 20,000 per 100,000, which is over 1,500 times higher than the actual U.S. suicide rate of 13 per 100,000— a very low prevalence. A reduction in the prevalence of suicide would not necessarily impact a scale's sensitivity and specificity, but it would have an enormous impact on the scale's overall accuracy. To put this into perspective, if we designed a nearly perfect suicide-risk screening scale that had 99% sensitivity (i.e., identified 99 out of 100 suicide decedents) and 99% specificity (i.e., identifies 99 out of 100 nonsuicide decedents) and then used it in a group of people with a suicide rate of 20,000 per 100,000, its positive predictive value would be 96%, meaning a positive screen on the scale would almost always be right. If that very same, nearly perfect scale were used to screen everyone in the United States, however, which has a much lower prevalence rate of 13 per 100,000, the positive predictive value would be 1.3%, meaning that a positive screen would almost always be wrong. Here again we have an apparent paradox: a nearly perfect scale can be wrong almost all the time when it's used in a population wherein the vast majority of individuals do *not* attempt suicide or die by suicide.

This is an important reality to recognize when advocating for universal suicide-risk screening—a common rallying cry of suicide prevention and mental health advocates. The best we can ever hope for in a suicide-risk screening tool designed to distinguish between those who will die by suicide and those who will not is being right only 1% of the time. The low accuracy of suicide-risk screening scales is a primary reason why various scientific bodies and clinician groups have resisted the suicide prevention community's call for wider implementation of suicide-risk screening, especially universal screening approaches intended to screen everyone on a regular basis. In 2004, for instance, the U.S. Preventative Services Task Force (USPSTF) was unable to find any studies showing that suicide-risk screening reduced suicide death or suicide attempts. Nearly a decade later, the USPSTF conducted another review of published research on suicide-risk screening and arrived at a similar conclusion: There was little evidence that routine screening in primary care medical settings could reliably identify patients with increased risk of attempting or dying by suicide.

In 2005, a separate team of researchers led by John Mann conducted a thorough review of suicide prevention strategies and concluded that although suicide-risk screening was associated with significant increases in identifying individuals who were thinking about suicide, no studies showed that screening led to reduced suicide attempts or deaths. This conclusion was bolstered by a 2017 study completed by Ivan Miller and colleagues examining how the implementation of routine suicide-risk screening in emergency departments could impact the probability of suicidal behaviors among patients during the following year. In Miller's study, routine screening of all patients who visited an emergency department for any reason had almost no impact on subsequent suicide attempt rates; reductions in suicidal behaviors didn't occur until a suicide-focused intervention was implemented.

Improving Suicide-Risk Screening and Detection

If suicide-risk screening has so many limitations, you might be wondering how we can identify those who are most at risk for suicide. If we don't know who's at risk, how will we be able to intervene to prevent suicide? To start, I think it's important to remember that knowing someone is (or is not) thinking about suicide is certainly better than not knowing, even if not by very much. When it comes to a wicked problem like suicide, though, thinking about suicide-risk screening in terms of "right or wrong" instead of "better or worse" is not especially meaningful. Second, it's also important to consider the possibility that suicide can be prevented without knowing for sure who will actually make a suicide attempt and who will not. We'll talk more about various strategies and measures for reducing suicidal behaviors in later chapters, but for the time being we can simply highlight that the assumption we must know who will attempt suicide in order to stop them from doing so makes about as much sense as saying that we need to know who is going to get into a car accident in order to prevent accidents from happening. There are almost certainly ways we can improve upon our current approach to suicide-risk screening and assessment that better align with the emergent nature of suicide risk. These better methods may have high error rates as well, but if the error rates are better than our current approaches, then that represents a net gain.

One possible approach informed by the concept of emergence involves methods that better capture the ever-changing nature of suicide risk and allow for complex, nonlinear relationships among the many variables that are associated with suicide. Methods that capture these two particular characteristics of emergence may be especially beneficial because one of the byproducts of emergence is change in temporal patterns, whereby a system's usual behavior shifts or otherwise alters when the system is about to undergo a state change. In many cases, increased dynamism is observed, meaning the system's typical change processes become more pronounced or vigorous. This process is depicted in Figure 3.5, which represents fluctuations in suicide risk over time for a hypothetical individual. In the left half of the figure,

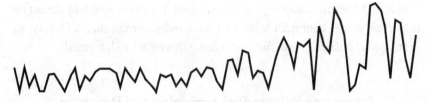

Figure 3.5 Increased dynamism in suicide risk fluctuations can involve larger magnitude fluctuations. For example, in the left hand portion of this figure, fluctuations in suicide risk are relatively small in magnitude but at around the midpoint these fluctuations become more pronounced and vigorous.

the individual's fluctuations in suicide risk are relatively mild, reflecting typical ups and downs. Starting at the midpoint, however, the fluctuations become increasingly pronounced, signaling a decline in self-regulation. After this point, the person finds it increasingly difficult to maintain balance in response to external forces.

To understand how this works, imagine a gymnast performing on the balance beam. To earn high marks in this event, gymnasts must be able to maintain their balance. They can do this by using a range of strategies such as repositioning their arms or legs, or otherwise shifting their weight in various ways to counteract the effects of gravity. In many cases, these adjustments and corrections are very slight, even imperceptible to those of us who are watching. If the gymnast loses her balance, however, these adjustments and corrections become more pronounced and apparent to us—the gymnast may wave her arms, bend her legs, and contort her body in extreme ways in an attempt to stabilize herself. With a combination of skill and luck, the gymnast will be able to self-correct and maintain her balance. In some cases, however, her self-corrections will not be enough and she will fall off the balance beam, thereby losing points. Falling off the balance beam marks the transition from one state (performing on the balance beam) to another state (being on the ground).

In Figure 3.6, fluctuations in suicide risk for a different hypothetical individual are displayed. In the left half of this figure, the fluctuations in suicide risk are relatively mild but there is an occasional spike. At around the midpoint, however, these spikes occur with much greater frequency. This is another way in which declining self-regulation might occur: increased frequency of a particular behavior. If we return to our balance beam example, a gymnast will occasionally shift her weight suddenly to maintain

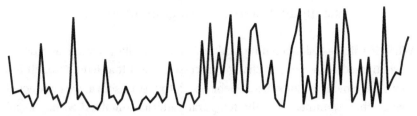

Figure 3.6 Increased dynamism in suicide risk fluctuations can also involve increased frequency of fluctuations. For example, in the left hand portion of this figure, large spikes in suicide risk occur with low frequency but at around the midpoint these spikes occur much more often.

balance. Anyone who has watched gymnastics can recall seeing the isolated but sudden repositioning of an arm or a hip thrown out to the side, each of which is designed to quickly regain balance. In most cases, these dramatic and extreme behaviors occur only infrequently during a given routine. When the gymnast is in jeopardy of falling off the beam, however, these extreme behaviors occur more frequently. The arm starts to wave up and down and the hips shift back and forth multiple times. Here again, a change pattern that is seen under typical conditions changes in a qualitatively distinct way: increased frequency. Under typical conditions, the self-corrections made by the gymnast are relatively small; under extreme conditions, however, those same self-corrections can become more extreme and more frequent. The changes observed in the movement of the gymnast's arms, legs, and torso during the time right before her fall can be understood as "warning signs," but if the gymnast regains her balance, they are instead "false alarms," so to speak.

Before a gymnastics meet begins, we cannot reliably predict which gymnasts are going to fall of the balance beam and which gymnasts are not. We also cannot reliably predict this outcome when the gymnast is walking up to the balance beam to begin her routine, even though a fall, if it happens, is only minutes (maybe even seconds) away. Even when we observe a gymnast suddenly waving her arms, bending her legs, repositioning her torso, and shifting her weight, we cannot always determine if the gymnast is going to fall or recover, but we do know that the probability of falling is significantly increased in that moment. In that moment, the gymnast is in a high-risk state. A fall won't happen every time the gymnast is in this high-risk state, but the probability of a fall is much, much higher.

Examining patterns of change in suicide risk

What if suicide-risk screening and assessment took a similar approach? If we focused on a person's change processes, could that tell us something about the emergence of suicidal behaviors? To test this idea, we conducted a study that examined how the temporal patterns contained within social media posts might signal the eventual emergence of suicidal behavior. In that study, we had a large team of students code the content of publicly accessible social media posts from 157 individuals who had died by suicide and 158 individuals who had died of nonsuicide causes. We then used a data analytic method based on the key assumptions of emergence: (1) change is constant; (2) the whole is greater than the sum of its parts; (3) each component of a system depends on the other components to function; and (4) complex systems behave in nonproportional ways. The results of this study indicated that individuals who died by suicide showed very different patterns of change over time than individuals who died of nonsuicide causes. Of note, the emergence of suicidal behavior was signaled by several changes in the usual patterns observed in a user's social media posts. One of the most prominent patterns involved coordinated change between social media posts describing negative thoughts or expectations and posts describing stressful life situations. Specifically, individuals who died by suicide tended to post content containing these two topics in close succession but individuals who died of nonsuicide causes did not. Expressing negative thoughts or expectations wasn't especially useful by itself, and neither were descriptions of stressful life situations, but when considered in combination, these two variables mattered a lot. This is what the third assumption of emergence would lead us to expect: The various components of a system depend on one another and cannot be understood in isolation.

We also found that some temporal patterns became more pronounced within individuals as the date of their death by suicide approached. As people got closer and closer to killing themselves, for instance, they were increasingly likely to post content describing stressful life situations followed by content describing negative thoughts or expectations. Here again, describing life situations and negative thoughts or expectations were not especially meaningful in isolation, but in combination they signaled the emergence of suicidal behavior. Interestingly, when we compared the social media content of individuals who died by suicide to the content of individuals who died of nonsuicide causes, there were minimal differences. Social media content did not, therefore, meaningfully distinguish *between* those who would eventually die by suicide and those who would not, but change in social media content *within* individuals signaled the approach of suicidal behavior, just as a gymnast's dramatic body movements can signal an approaching fall but the same body movements across multiple gymnasts may not be so helpful in determining who will fall and who will not.

Not long after we first presented these results at the annual conference of the American Association of Suicidology, a team of researchers led by Kate Loveys applied a version of this concept, which they called "micropatterns," to data obtained from users of the Twitter social media platform. Their results indicated that the examination of micropatterns—in other words, considering how change among multiple variables depended on one another—provided a significant boost in identifying users who had attempted suicide. Interestingly, Loveys's team referred to these micropatterns as "small but mighty," a descriptor that fits nicely with the fourth assumption of emergence involving nonproportional behavior: Small change can lead to big differences in outcomes.

Within the past few years, we've also applied the concepts of emergence to test their utility when used in clinical settings. To do this, we asked 28 patients who had previously attempted suicide to rate the intensity of their suicidal thoughts during the past week at the start of each therapy session. Because these therapy sessions were typically scheduled one week apart, we were able to examine how weekly fluctuations in suicidal thinking were related to the eventual emergence of suicidal behaviors. We first analyzed the data using traditional methods designed to distinguish between those who eventually attempted suicide again and those who did not, but this approach was unsuccessful: Intensity of suicidal ideation failed to distinguish the two groups. Next, we analyzed the data using a method based on the concepts of emergence. When we conducted these second analyses we did not find that change in suicidal ideation differed between those patients who attempted suicide and those who did not, but change in suicidal ideation within individuals was qualitatively different for those who eventually attempted suicide. Specifically, the pattern we saw was similar to the pattern displayed in Figure 3.6: more frequent and more rapid ups and downs.

The gymnast who is fighting to keep her balance on the balance beam has a much higher probability of falling than the gymnast who is balanced and calm. When a given gymnast's behavior changes in particular ways, the accuracy of our predictions regarding the probability of that particular gymnast falling is increased considerably. Our accuracy would be reduced, however, if we tried to predict which of multiple flailing gymnasts were going to fall and which were not. In like fashion, our estimation of an individual's risk for attempting suicide may be improved when we consider how their change patterns are deviating from *their own typical patterns*, but our accuracy is reduced when we try to distinguish between those who will attempt suicide and those who will not. Taken together, these results suggest that suicide-risk screening and assessment may be improved by repeatedly assessing various indicators of suicide risk over time and being alert for certain types of departures from an individual's typical change pattern. This shift in perspective is probably most relevant for mental health clinicians who can repeatedly assess and monitor suicidal thinking and other potential indicators of suicide risk such as mood, sleep, and hopelessness, over the course of treatment.

This particular approach may be less useful in certain medical settings such as emergency departments and primary care clinics, however, where patient visits are more likely to be infrequent and/or episodic. In settings like these, alternative methods such as machine learning and artificial intelligence may be more valuable. These computationally intensive methods are able to combine a whole bunch of variables and examine lots of different combinations and configurations of these variables to identify the optimal values for each. Machine learning methods have advanced rapidly over the past few years and hold considerable promise for suicide-risk screening and assessment because they can consider very complex combinations of variables, thereby capitalizing upon the second and third assumptions of emergence.

An interesting finding from machine-learning-based studies is that many risk factors and correlates of suicide are not necessarily elevated or extreme in the resulting algorithms. In other words, individuals with severe levels of depression, hopelessness, anxiety, and other similar risk factors may not actually carry the highest risk for suicidal behaviors; individuals with moderate or even low levels of these variables may, in some cases, carry the highest risk for suicide. This departs from our historic assumption that suicide occurs as a result of extreme levels of these (and other) risk factors. When it comes to wicked problems such as suicide, however, this assumption doesn't have to be true; it's entirely possible that the optimal combination of these variables is something along the lines of moderate depression combined with low anxiety combined with severe hopelessness combined with any amount of suicidal ideation. Because suicide is indeterminate, there also may be other combinations of these same variables that are less optimal but nonetheless work; just as the equation $X + Y = 10$ can be true if $X = 10$ and $Y = 0$ or if $X = 5$ and $Y = 5$ or if $X = -57$ and $Y = 67$, there can potentially be multiple "correct" combinations of suicide risk and protective factors, including combinations that do not include indicators of mental illness at all. Some of these combinations may be better than other combinations, but it wouldn't be accurate to use the terms "right" or "correct" to describe these combinations.

As compared to more traditional methods of suicide-risk screening, newer algorithms based on machine learning methods have provided better sensitivity and specificity, but their overall accuracy remains limited because even the most sophisticated algorithms are not immune to the effects of low prevalence. Machine learning algorithms, therefore, have very high false positive rates, such that a positive screen is correct in fewer than 1 out of 100 cases, on average. Machine learning algorithms, therefore, may be more useful for identifying *subgroups* within which risk is highly concentrated as opposed to identifying high-risk *individuals*. This approach is akin to how the meteorologist forecasts which communities and regions are likely to experience dangerous weather conditions despite an inability to reliably forecast or predict which specific buildings and homes will be damaged by a tornado or another severe weather event. Indeed, meteorologists don't waste much time trying to determine whose homes will be damaged and whose homes will not be damaged, and we don't expect them to be able to do this even though such predictions would be very popular and highly valued.

When it comes to protecting ourselves and our homes from weather-related damages, we have the benefit of many, many decades of research focused on improving weather forecasting methods. Suicide research, by comparison, is a much newer (and therefore younger) enterprise. Hundreds of years ago, weather forecasting was crude and rudimentary. Today, weather forecasting is remarkably accurate, even though it cannot tell us which homes will be damaged and which will not. Our thinking about suicide-risk screening and assessment could potentially benefit a great deal by following a similar course. Specifically, we should move away from assuming that we must know who will and who will not attempt suicide to prevent these behaviors from occurring. Indeed, we could prevent suicides even without knowing who is most likely to make a suicide attempt; and we will discuss this point in greater depth in later chapters. We also need to abandon any expectation that suicide-risk screening will ever be able to achieve the level of precision and accuracy that we desire, and think instead about how we could develop better methods for identifying and intervening with individuals whose probability for suicide has increased because they are about to shift to a high-risk state.

4

Performance Escapes and Catastrophes

Suicide risk constantly changes. As we discussed in the previous chapter, in some cases this change can occur very rapidly and suddenly. In Kleiman's ecological momentary assessment (EMA) study, for instance, 9 out of 10 participants experienced a large shift in suicidal ideation within only a few hours. The Marine I met with in Iraq certainly experienced this: In less than one hour he moved from a status quo state, to experiencing his first-ever thoughts about suicide, to placing an M16 under his chin and pulling the trigger. "It just happened," he said, unable to explain his behavior in the absence of any obvious precipitating event or change in circumstances. The patient who suddenly grabbed his firearm during an argument with his wife described a similar rapid shift in risk level and provided a similar explanation: "It just happened." Kleiman's results and the Marine's sudden suicide attempt each speak to the fourth assumption of emergence: Complex systems behave in nonproportional ways. Relatively small changes can therefore lead to drastically different outcomes and, conversely, relatively large changes can seem to have no effect on outcomes whatsoever. This is part of the reason why suicide warning signs and suicide-risk screening tools are much less precise than we would like.

Why do some suicides seem to occur "out of the blue," without much (or any) advance warning, whereas other suicides seem much less surprising? How can someone seem to be doing OK, right up to the point of making a suicide attempt? Is it possible for suicide to occur without any warning signs? These questions reflect the traditional assumption that change in suicide-risk level reflects a unidimensional continuum, akin to that depicted in Figure 4.1. According to this traditional continuum model, suicide risk is understood to be a spectrum that is anchored on the lower end by the absence of thoughts about death or suicide and on the upper end by suicidal behavior. Between these extremes are various types of suicidal thoughts and intentions. This unidimensional suicide-risk continuum serves as the basis for most, if not all, of the recommended strategies for preventing suicide. Suicidal thoughts are, for instance, assumed to be a necessary precondition for suicidal behavior,

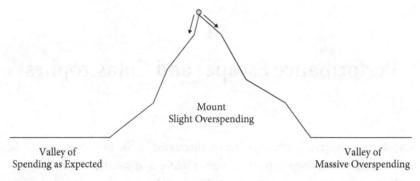

Figure 4.1 NASA project spending behavior can be represented topologically to understand how performance escapes emerge over time. Spending as expected and massive overspending are represented by two valleys separated by a mountain peak, which corresponds to the tipping point contained within slight overspending. Project spending at any given time corresponds to the location of the ball along the horizontal: as the ball moves from left to right, project spending increases. If the ball is kicked towards the mountain from the Valley of Spending as Expected, it will likely roll partway up the mountain slope, slow down and stop, then roll back to the valley floor. If the ball is kicked with enough force, however, it could reach the peak of the mountain. If it crosses over the mountain peak, it will start rolling down the opposite side of the mountain towards the Valley of Massive Overspending. Because of gravity, the ball will not spend much time on Mount Slight Overspending. Performance escapes work in a similar manner. If a project is slightly overspending but does not pass over the tipping point, project spending reverses course and returns to spending as expected. If a project that is slightly overspending passes the tipping point, however, project spending rapidly increases, leading to performance escape.

serving as the gateway through which one must pass to get to suicidal behavior. Different types of suicidal thoughts are further assumed to fall along different points along this suicide-risk continuum. Serious suicidal ideation (e.g., "I want to kill myself") is located above the wish for death (e.g., "I wish I were dead") because the former is assumed to be a stronger indicator of one's propensity to engage in suicidal behavior than the latter. Likewise, suicide planning, which entails specific thoughts about how, when, and where one will attempt suicide, is located above serious suicidal ideation. Because an individual's location on the suicide-risk continuum is assumed to reflect his or her propensity to eventually engage in suicidal behaviors, suicide-risk screening and assessment methods often focus on asking individuals to disclose or endorse various qualities of their suicidal thoughts (e.g., frequency of suicidal thoughts, intensity of suicidal thoughts), which can then be used to estimate their location on the continuum, with individuals located higher on the continuum deemed "higher risk" because they are assumed to be more likely to make a suicide attempt or die by suicide.

Despite the general acceptance of this unidimensional suicide-risk continuum by researchers and clinicians, a considerable body of research suggests this perspective may be less useful than traditionally assumed. Numerous studies have found, for instance, that around half of individuals who attempt suicide deny serious suicidal ideation, suicide planning, and/or preparatory or rehearsal behaviors[1] in the time leading up to their attempt. In a study conducted by Marianne Wyder and Diego De Leo, two out of three individuals who were interviewed soon after they had attempted suicide denied experiencing one or more of these intermediate levels of the suicide-risk continuum. In this study, six out of 10 individuals who attempted suicide said they did not make any plans or arrangements to take their lives prior to attempting suicide, three out of 10 reported they did not seriously consider taking their own life, and two out of 10 reported they did not think about taking their lives at all. Approximately half of U.S. adults who have attempted suicide similarly deny they had made a plan in advance.

If suicide risk existed on a unidimensional continuum, we would expect that most (if not all) individuals who transition from lower to higher levels of suicide risk would also experience these intermediate levels of suicide risk as part of the transition from lower to higher risk states. Individuals who have attempted suicide give us a very different picture, however: Most (if not all) were previously in a low risk state but only half experienced intermediate risk states, almost as if they had skipped over these intervening risk levels. This suggests that, at least for some people, suicide risk may not lie on a unidimensional spectrum or continuum. Rather, two distinct states seem to exist, one that is low risk and one that is high risk, sort of like two buckets placed side by side. Under these circumstances, changes in suicide risk would take the character of sudden jumps from one state to the other rather than the smooth, gradual transition that characterizes the unidimensional continuum.

Because of nonproportionality—the fourth key assumption of emergence—change can sometimes be both smooth or continuous and other times be sudden and jarring, almost as if it came out of the blue. Both are possible, but only if we move beyond the unidimensional continuum model of suicide risk.

Performance Escapes

In the world of dynamical systems, sudden and discontinuous change processes are often referred to as "catastrophic" change because they represent a fundamental shift in how a system operates. Catastrophic change can be so dramatic that it defies reason and can't be easily anticipated; up until the catastrophic change occurs, there is little to no indication that the change is even possible (sounds just like suicide, doesn't it?) Indeed, the destructive impact of catastrophic change processes is almost entirely due to their apparent unpredictability.

As with emergence in general, I learned about catastrophic change processes from Jon Butner. Jon introduced me to the concept of catastrophic change while he and I were talking about the projects that each of us was working on for the National Aeronautics and Space Administration (NASA). I had been asked to provide recommendations for assessing and monitoring the psychological and behavioral health of astronauts returning from long-duration space flight missions (manned missions to Mars, for example), and Jon had been asked to develop mathematical models for identifying projects with "performance escapes," a term that refers to projects that suddenly start to vastly overspend their planned budgets. Performance escapes had an out-of-the-blue quality, seemingly occurring with little to no advance warning; these projects would be progressing well for months or even years before suddenly shifting to massive overspending. Luckily, performance escapes didn't happen very often, but their consequences tended to be disproportionately large because they negatively impacted the budgets and operations of so many different offices and divisions, potentially leading to downstream problems and delays across multiple projects. A single performance escape project could therefore create major problems for a whole lot of people.

To understand how performance escapes suddenly emerged from otherwise successful projects, Jon focused on how the spending behavior of a project changed over time so he could identify deviations from the norm. He did not, however, attempt to measure all of the many risk factors that might be correlated with spending behavior, such as size of the project team, nature of the project objectives, or past performance of the team. I was surprised to learn this, because that's how I would have approached the problem. I would have assessed and quantified as many variables as possible and then constructed some sort of statistical model to identify the "right" combination of these many variables that best distinguished performance escapes from every other project. Note that this is how suicide risk has typically been studied. Such an approach assumes that performance escapes are a conventional problem that can be definitively "solved" by identifying and modifying the "right" strategies. Performance escapes are not a conventional problem, though; they are a wicked problem. As a systems-informed researcher, Jon recognized this and took a very different approach. He did not attempt to identify the characteristics of performance escape projects and differentiate them from the characteristics of other projects. Instead, he sought to determine what might signal when a particular project was about to move off course and switch from an on-track project to a performance escape. Said another way, Jon was looking for the financial equivalent of flailing arms, legs, and torsos that occur right before a gymnast falls off the balance beam.

When Jon had finished his analyses, his results indicated that there were three "types" of projects: (1) those that were on budget for the duration of the project, (2) those that were significantly over budget for the duration of the project, and (3) those that started on budget but suddenly switched to being significantly over budget. The first project type was not of concern to NASA for obvious reasons: These were the "ideal" projects that managers hoped for and aspired to. The second project type was characterized by consistent over-spending from the very beginning; they started over budget and remained over budget. Interestingly, these projects were not of much concern either, which surprised me until I understood the rationale: even though these projects were significantly over budget, they were *consistently* over budget. Because these projects overspent from the start and continued to overspend across the entire project, they were stable and predictable, so there wasn't much uncertainty surrounding them. Managers could, therefore, fairly easily design and implement solutions that would protect the rest of the organization from the effects of their predictable overspending. Sure, on-budget spending was preferred, but if a project is going to overspend, overspending in a predictable way was strongly preferred to overspending in an unpredictable way.

This unpredictability was the hallmark characteristic of the third project type, the performance escape. In these projects, things started off OK—projects were generally spending as planned or only slightly more than expected—but then suddenly they started spending like mad. Most frustratingly, there seemed to be no way to distinguish these projects from the first project type, those that started and stayed on budget. This third project type, therefore, carried the greatest amount of uncertainty and the greatest amount of risk; it seemed to be doing OK right up until the point that it suddenly was not. Compounding the problem was the fact that there was no way of knowing in advance which projects would become performance escapes and when this shift to massive overspending would occur.

Jon's results further indicated that although three types of projects existed, there were only two general patterns of spending behavior: (1) spending at the expected level or (2) overspending at a rate that was, on average, around four times higher than the expected rate. In other words, projects either spent $1 for every expected $1 or they spent $4 (on average) for every expected $1. Although massive overspending was reasonably common, slight overspending along the lines of $1.20 or $1.50 for every expected $1 did not occur very often, and moderate overspending—along the lines of $2 or $2.50 for every expected $1—occurred even less often. In fact, a moderate amount of overspending was so exceedingly rare that it practically didn't exist at all. When slight overspending occurred on a project, one of two things tended to happen soon thereafter: Spending either reduced, returning to expected spending levels, or it dramatically increased, resulting in a rapid shift to massive overspending. A "tipping point" of sorts, therefore, existed somewhere in the realm of slight overspending. If project spending reached this tipping point and moved past it, even if only very slightly, spending would suddenly increase by a very large amount. Once spending reached this level, the project rarely reversed course, resulting in performance escape. A relatively small change in spending from one time period to the next, therefore, led to an enormously disproportionate outcome—the hallmark of catastrophic change.

Tipping Points

In dynamical systems theory, tipping points implicate the existence of multiple stable states that are qualitatively different from one another. In the case of NASA project spending, there were two stable states of spending: spending as expected (e.g., $1 for every expected $1) and massively overspending (e.g., $4 for every expected $1). NASA projects were very likely to behave in one of these two ways. Slight overspending (e.g., $1.50 for every expected $1), by comparison, occurred much less often and generally did not last for very long, and moderate overspending (e.g., $2 to $2.50 for every expected $1) was almost unheard of. Once a project reached this level of slight-to-moderate overspending, it rarely stayed in this state: the project either self-corrected or it got much, much worse.

To understand how this works, imagine two valleys separated by a mountain range (see Figure 4.1). If we were to place a ball on the peak of the mountain, it would roll down one side of the mountain or the other, to one of the two valleys below, but it's very unlikely that the ball would remain motionless on the very tip of the peak. The two valleys correspond to the two spending patterns identified in Jon's NASA study—spending as expected and massive overspending—and the mountain peak corresponds to the tipping point associated with slight or moderate overspending. Just as a ball placed on the peak of the mountain would quickly roll down one side of the mountain or the other, slight-to-moderate overspending on a NASA project quickly gravitated toward one of the two stable spending patterns: spending as expected or massive overspending.

Now imagine that we place a ball on the ground in the Valley of Spending as Expected. This is where all NASA projects start: spending as expected. If a ball located in this valley is kicked toward Mount Slight Overspending, one of two things will happen. The first possibility is for the ball to fall short of the peak and roll back down the slope to the floor of the Valley of Spending as Expected. If the ball is kicked with enough force, however, the second option is for the ball to pass over the peak of Mount Slight Overspending and roll down to the opposite valley. The first possibility is observed in the first and third project types. For the first project type, the ball always remains in the Valley of Spending as Expected; no matter how many times it is kicked toward the mountain, it falls short of the peak and rolls back down to spending as expected. This is also how things go during the outset of the third project type (performance escapes). The first possibility, therefore, is observed only in the first and third project types.

The second possibility—kicking the ball over the mountain so that it ends up in the Valley of Massive Overspending, is observed only in the second and third project types. For the second project type, the ball passes over the mountain peak and rolls down to the Valley of Massive Overspending very early on. Unfortunately, because there's no one in the Valley of Massive Overspending who can kick the ball back over the mountain, the ball remains in that valley indefinitely. For the third project type (performance escapes), this process happens as well, but only after the ball has been in the Valley of Spending as Expected for a much longer period of time. No matter how the ball is kicked, the ball will not spend much time on either the peak of the mountain or on the mountain's slopes because gravity will pull the ball down toward one of the valley floors. The ball will therefore spend most of its time in one of the valleys. To kick the ball from one valley to the other would require a lot of force and momentum. As such, the movement from one valley to the other would seem sudden and unexpected, possibly taking us off guard.

As I learned more about Jon's project, I was struck by the many parallels between performance escapes and suicide. People often appeared to be doing OK, then suddenly they were dead, seemingly without warning. Also similar to project escapes, suicides occur infrequently, but their consequences can be enormous, especially for the family and broader community. These consequences often take the form of increased health problems for loss survivors; financial costs associated with medical treatment, social services, and funeral arrangements; and economic consequences resulting from lost productivity. Suicide and performance escapes have another similarity: Both are affected by a dizzying array of factors and variables, all of which impact and influence one another. In the case of performance escapes, these factors could include things such as the nature of the project objectives, size of the project team, turnover of project team members, fluctuations in travel and material costs, and more. In the case of suicide, these factors could include things such as mood state, financial status, access to health care, genetic and biological predispositions, and more. Attempting to measure all of the variables that may be relevant to both performance escapes and suicide would be impossible. Performance escapes and suicide, therefore, cannot be comprehensively explained with a single, definitive model or problem definition, and no single solution or combination of solutions can be considered "right" or "correct," even though some solutions may be relatively better than others.

I was especially intrigued by the tipping point notion. Like performance escapes, individuals who died by suicide often seemed to be doing reasonably well right up until the moment they were attempting suicide, as if they had crossed over some sort of threshold or tipping point. The notion of a tipping point not only aligned with my own observations of suicidal patients and the experiences of suicide loss survivors; it also aligned with the subjective experience of many patients I had treated over the years. Many (though not all) of my patients often said that they didn't necessarily feel any better or any worse than they had the day before (or the week or the month before that). On the contrary, they often explained that they "just couldn't take it anymore," implying that they had crossed some boundary that lies between attempting suicide and not. When I would ask these patients what had changed in the time leading up to their attempt, they often couldn't identify a precipitating event or point to a particular reason. "I don't know," many of them said. "It just happened." A relatively small change—a slight nudge—had effectively pushed them past this tipping point, resulting in a catastrophic outcome. With Jon's help and guidance, I therefore started researching catastrophe models.

Implications for Suicide

Various catastrophe models have been identified and described, typically by mathematicians, but one model in particular, known as the *cusp catastrophe model*, has proven to be especially useful in a wide range of fields and disciplines including biology, physics, economics, and management. The cusp catastrophe model was the type Jon used to describe the spending behavior of NASA performance escapes. The cusp catastrophe model is characterized by five specific properties: (1) the system has two distinct states; (2) change between these two states occurs suddenly; (3) certain states are highly improbable; (4) very small changes in conditions can lead to very different outcomes; and (5) the conditions under which a transition from one state to the other occurs do not necessarily coincide with the conditions under which a transition occurs in the opposite direction. If applied to suicide risk, we arrive at the five properties summarized in Box 4.1.

Box 4.1. Five Properties of the Cusp Catastrophe Model of Suicide

---

1. Suicide risk has two distinct states.
2. Change between suicide-risk states occurs suddenly.
3. Certain suicide-risk states are highly improbable.
4. Very small changes in risk and protective factors can lead to very different outcomes in suicide risk, specifically, attempting suicide or not.
5. The conditions under which someone transitions from low suicide risk to high suicide risk do not necessarily coincide with the conditions under which someone transitions from high suicide risk to low suicide risk.

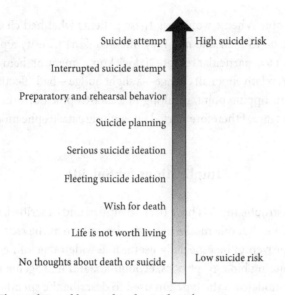

Figure 4.2 The traditional hierarchical suicide risk continuum.

The cusp catastrophe model stands in contrast to the unidimensional suicide-risk continuum model that has dominated thinking about suicide risk for decades and is depicted in Figure 4.2., a pattern that mirrors what Jon found in his NASA research: Spending was either on budget or massively over budget; it was almost never between these two extremes.

Suicide risk is characterized by two distinct states

The existence of two distinct suicide-risk states is further bolstered by studies using a data analytic method called *taxometric analysis*. Taxometric analysis is a statistical procedure that can help researchers determine if multiple things belong to a single group or if they belong to different groups. In the case of suicide risk, taxometric analysis can be used to determine if different types of suicidal thoughts, behaviors, and associated symptoms of mental illness are best understood as existing along the unidimensional suicide-risk continuum or if they belong to separate, distinct groups. In the first study to use this method, Tracy Witte and Jill Holm-Denoma analyzed the survey responses of 1,773 U.S. military personnel and veterans and in the second study, Katrina Rufino analyzed the responses of 2,385 patients who had been hospitalized for suicide risk. In both studies, results suggested that suicide risk was comprised of two distinct subgroups—one low risk and one high risk—rather than existing on a unidimensional continuum. Both studies also found that the differences between the two subgroups were most pronounced for variables directly related to suicide risk, such as severity and intensity of suicidal thoughts. Differences between the high-risk and the low-risk groups, by comparison, were very small when considering variables such as depression, hopelessness, and other symptoms of mental illness. The subgroup characterized by more severe suicidal thoughts also had a much higher percentage of participants who had previously attempted suicide. Furthermore, symptoms of mental illness did not meaningfully distinguish these two subgroups.[2]

Yet another line of evidence comes from a study of over 40,000 U.S. Army Soldiers who had been hospitalized for reasons related to psychological or emotional distress, to include elevated suicide risk. In that study, researchers from the Army Study to Assess Risk and Resilience in Servicemembers (Army STARRS) developed a risk algorithm using machine learning methods to identify subgroups of military personnel with very high rates of suicide death. Twenty subgroups comprised of almost 2,700 Soldiers each were identified by the algorithm and rank ordered according to the number of suicide deaths within each subgroup. Of the 68 Soldiers who died by suicide during the year after being discharged from the hospital, 36 (i.e., just over half of all the suicides) belonged to a single subgroup. The remaining 32 suicides were distributed across all of the remaining subgroups (see the left panel of Figure 4.3). If suicide risk existed on a continuum, we would expect to see a much more gradual change in the number of suicides across subgroups, perhaps something along the lines of the distribution plotted in the right panel of Figure 4.3. We don't, of course, see this pattern at all. Instead, we see a big difference between the first subgroup and every other subgroup—along with minimal differences among the remaining 19 subgroups. Two discrete subgroups are therefore implicated: one that is high risk (i.e., Subgroup 1) and one that is low risk (i.e., Subgroups 2 through 20). In combination, these three studies lend support to the first and third properties of the cusp catastrophe model: Suicide risk has two distinct states and intermediate suicide risk levels are much less probable than lower and higher risk levels.

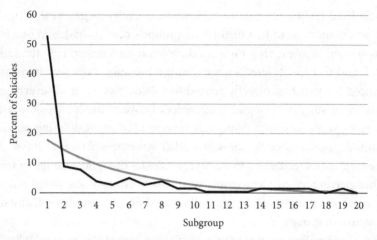

Figure 4.3 In a sample of over 40,000 U.S. Soldiers, researchers used a machine learning risk algorithm to sort Soldiers into one of 20 subgroups of 2,700 Soldiers each. As shown by the black line, one of the 20 subgroups included more than half of all the suicide deaths. This pattern supports the existence of two distinct suicide risk states, one that is high risk and one that is low risk. If suicide risk existed on a hierarchical continuum, the distribution of suicide deaths across the 20 subgroups would have looked closer to the grey line. (Source: Kessler et al., 2015)

Change between suicide-risk states can occur suddenly

Multiple lines of evidence also support the second property of the cusp catastrophe model: Change between suicide-risk states occurs suddenly. Indeed, we've known for decades that the shift from low-risk to high-risk states can occur very rapidly. Back in 1980, for instance, Christopher Williams and colleagues found that almost half (four out of 10) individuals who attempted suicide reported making the decision to do so with less than five minutes of advance deliberation. Similar results have subsequently been reported by multiple research teams, suggesting that up to half of suicide attempts occur within five to 20 minutes of deliberation over the act. A recent study by Alex Millner and colleagues provides what is arguably the most nuanced understanding to date of how fast this transition can occur. In that study, Millner interviewed 30 individuals who had recently attempted suicide and asked these individuals to reflect upon their experiences leading up to the attempt. On average, participants reported the following timeline:

- Five years prior to the attempt, they first experienced suicidal thoughts and experienced these thoughts off and on for several years;
- Two weeks prior to the attempt, these suicidal thoughts increased in intensity and frequency, such that they were occurring nearly continuously;
- One week prior to the attempt, they started to think about where to attempt suicide;
- Six hours prior to the attempt, they experienced an internal debate about whether or not to attempt suicide;
- Two hours prior to the attempt, they decided upon which method to use;
- Thirty minutes prior to the attempt, they decided where to make the attempt; and
- Five minutes prior to the attempt, they made the final decision to act.

Millner mathematically modeled the temporal progression through these steps and showed that the process of transitioning from low-risk to high-risk states was exponential instead of linear, which means that individuals accelerated through these various steps rapidly, within a very brief window of time, rather than incrementally or gradually. For most individuals, suicidal thinking remained relatively low in intensity until just a few hours before making the attempt, at which point the progression toward suicidal behavior rapidly accelerated. Because of this rapid change, individuals spent only a very brief period of time in the intermediate-risk levels, suggesting that many individuals who deny experiencing intermediate levels of risk in the time leading up to their suicide attempts may not have skipped these levels completely, but traversed them so quickly that they weren't noticed.

Certain levels of suicide risk are uncommon

Milner's results further suggest that suicidal mulling, a psychological state during which an individual experiences an internal debate about whether or not to make the suicide attempt, may serve as the tipping point between low-risk and high-risk states. Before individuals reach this point, thoughts about suicide remain relatively mild and low risk, but after passing this point, individuals very quickly move from ideation to action. If people reach this state of suicidal mulling but do not cross over the tipping point, they will return to a low-risk state. If, however, they pass the threshold of this tipping point, they will rapidly transition to a high-risk state. While in a state of suicidal mulling, the very slightest of nudges in either direction could make the difference between returning to a lower risk state or transitioning to a higher risk state where the probability of suicidal behavior is greatly increased.

This gives rise to the third property of the cusp catastrophe model: Certain states are highly improbable. As discussed earlier in this chapter, states characterized by severe levels of suicidal ideation and/or suicidal planning are the likeliest levels to be "skipped" by people in the time leading up to their suicide attempts. One possibility is that people truly are not experiencing these levels of suicide risk at all. Another possibility is that people do experience these levels of suicide risk but spend such little time in these states that they are missed or unrecognized. In either case, people generally do not spend much time in these intermediate-risk states; they pass through or leave soon after arriving.

Small changes in suicide risk can lead to (very) big differences

The tipping point between two discrete suicide-risk states provides the basis for the fourth property of the cusp catastrophe model: Very small changes in conditions can lead to very different outcomes. If this property sounds familiar, that's because it is also one of the key assumptions of emergence: nonproportionality. As applied to suicide, nonproportionality means that a very small change could push an individual who is debating about whether or not to attempt suicide in one direction or the other. Likewise, two individuals who are similar to each other may nonetheless display very different outcomes: one might die by suicide while the other does not, for instance. Under the right conditions, the smallest of changes to one person but not the other could result in different outcomes. Conversely, when someone is *not* at the tipping point, very large changes in stress could have hardly any impact on their suicide-risk level.

One of the clearest demonstrations of this principle comes from a study published by Greg Brown in 2005. In that study, Brown examined how the balance between the wish to live and the wish to die, two competing drives that align with Millner's concept of "mulling," was associated with eventual suicide. Brown compared patients' responses on a three-point scale that asked them to rate how strongly they wanted to live and a three-point scale that asked them to rate how strongly they wanted to die. Brown then subtracted each patient's wish to live score from their wish to die score, resulting in a score that essentially quantified each person's balance between the wish to live and the wish to die. Patients who had a very strong wish to die combined with no wish to live—the highest score possible—were more than six times more likely to die by suicide than everyone else. Among patients who had at least *some* wish to live, however, the risk of suicide was significantly reduced, suggesting that even a small wish to live could offset a whole lot of wish to die. Conversely, a relatively small decline in the wish to live could precipitate the emergence of suicidal behavior.

Indeed, this is what we found in a study published with my colleagues in 2016. We asked suicidal individuals to rate their wish to live and their wish to die every few months over the course of two years. We found that relatively small decreases in the wish to live were associated with the emergence of suicidal behaviors, but change in the wish to die—even large change—was not. When it comes to the tipping point between suicidal behavior and the absence of it, the wish to live seems to carry somewhat more weight than the wish to die.

Becoming suicidal and recovering from suicidal states do not mirror each other

This brings us to the fifth and final property of the cusp catastrophe model: The change process in one direction is not always mirrored by the change process in the opposite direction. As applied to suicide risk, this suggests that the process of increasing suicide risk may differ from the process of decreasing suicide risk. If we want to move someone from a high-risk state to a low-risk state—a common goal of many suicide prevention interventions and treatments—simply "undoing" or reversing the conditions under which they became suicidal may not be enough. Returning to gymnastics, a gymnast who has fallen off the balance beam cannot get back up by waving her arms and legs around and shifting her weight back and forth, even though these things happened right before she fell. She must instead engage in a completely different set of behaviors—lifting herself up, for instance—to resume her routine.

The technical term for this property is *hysteresis,* and refers to the fact that a system's current state depends on the system's previous state. Said another way: history matters. Change will follow different pathways that are shaped by the system's past. To understand hysteresis, think about how memory foam behaves. If you sit on a memory foam pillow, it will change shape almost immediately to conform to your body's contour. After you stand up again, the memory foam will expand and recover its original shape, but this expansion process will be much slower and take much longer than the compression process. When being compressed, memory foam rapidly changes but when expanding in the opposite direction, memory foam changes much more slowly. Change in one direction therefore does not mirror change in the opposite direction. Over time, as you sit on the memory foam pillow many times, it will gradually preserve its compressed shape, such that it stops expanding so much after you get up. This is how memory foam "remembers" its shape. With enough time, memory foam will preserve this shape that it takes when compressed, such that it changes very little at all. Here again, history matters; memory foam "remembers" its shape only after it has been compressed many times. If we wanted to understand the behavior of memory foam, we would therefore need to know two things: (1) the current state of the memory foam (is it currently compressed or not?) and (2) the history of the memory foam (how many times has it been compressed?).

The concept of hysteresis implicates the possibility that the process of *becoming* suicidal and the process of *recovering* from a suicidal state are not necessarily mirror images of each other. High-risk states can emerge rapidly, but returning to a low-risk state may take much longer. Hysteresis also provides a way to understand why a person's suicide risk can be so dramatically increased in the weeks and months after they have been discharged from an inpatient psychiatric facility. The degree of this increased risk is staggering: Someone who has been psychiatrically hospitalized is more than 100 times more likely than someone who has never been hospitalized to die by suicide. This risk is highest in the weeks immediately following discharge and slowly declines over time, but remains elevated even a year after discharge. This slow, gradual decline in suicide risk after hospitalization stands in stark contrast to the rapid rise in suicide risk that precipitated the hospitalization in the first place. Someone can move from low risk to high risk very rapidly but take months or years to move back to a low-risk state.

What's most remarkable about the incredibly high risk for suicide after someone has been discharged from inpatient hospitalization is that the discharge often occurs soon after a mental health professional determines that the person's suicide risk is no longer elevated. A colleague once observed wryly that the most reliable correlate of suicide after leaving a psychiatric in-patient unit is having been assessed by a mental health professional who has determined that a patient's suicide risk has decreased. The concept of hyster-esis suggests that although an individual's risk level when they are leaving the hospital may be lower than it was when they arrived, this reduction may not actually reflect a full return to a low-risk state.

Some have argued that this elevated risk for suicide immediately following discharge points to inpatient psychiatric treatment as a harmful practice. This is undoubtedly true for some—maybe many—individuals who are hospital-ized, but it's not true for everyone; I'm aware of plenty of people who have benefited from psychiatric hospitalization. I think a better explanation for the incredibly high suicide rate after psychiatric hospitalization is hysteresis. Just as memory foam quickly compresses under pressure but slowly recovers after the pressure has been removed, suicidal individuals may quickly transi-tion from a low-risk to high-risk state when under pressure but experience a much slower recovery after that pressure has been removed.

A Cusp Catastrophe Model of Suicide

To see how these five properties of suicide risk are related to one another, a three-dimensional cusp catastrophe model of suicide risk is depicted in Figure 4.4. In this figure, suicide risk is represented by the vertical axis, such that more severe levels of suicide risk are located above less severe levels. This part of the model is unchanged from the traditional unidimensional suicide-risk continuum model depicted previously in Figure 4.2, although I should clarify that, in this model, "suicide risk" represents the probability of making a suicide attempt. In contrast to the older model, which represents all pos-sible manifestations of suicide risk on a one-dimensional line, the cusp catas-trophe model of suicide risk represents all possible manifestations of suicide risk along a three-dimensional sheet called the "behavior surface." Regions of the behavior sheet with a higher altitude correspond to higher risk states, whereas regions of the sheet with a lower altitude correspond to lower risk states. Consistent with this convention, the lowest possible risk state (i.e., having no suicidal thoughts) is located in the lowest region of the behavior surface and the highest risk state (i.e., making a suicide attempt) is located in the highest region of the behavior surface. Moving "downhill" along the be-havior surface therefore corresponds to a reduction in suicide risk, whereas

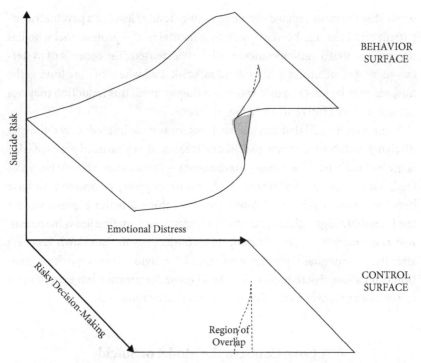

Figure 4.4 A topological depiction of suicide risk based on the cusp catastrophe model, wherein the probability of making a suicide attempt increases as one rises up the suicide risk axis.

moving "uphill" along the behavior surface corresponds to an increase in suicide risk.

Underneath the behavior surface is the control surface, which represents all of the possible combinations of two variables that are called control parameters. Control parameters are so named because they determine or influence the shape of the behavior surface, including the location and size of the double fold that you can see in the behavior surface. This double fold is central to understanding catastrophic change processes. We'll return to this important feature shortly. In the cusp catastrophe model of suicide depicted in Figure 4.4, the two control parameters that we'll consider are emotional distress and decision-making style. Emotional distress runs from left to right and decision-making style runs from back to front. I selected emotional distress as one of the two control parameters for reasons that are probably obvious: An abundant literature exists showing that various forms of emotional distress, broadly defined, are positively correlated with suicide risk. I want to clarify that emotional distress, as used here, does not necessarily mean mental illness per se; mental illness and its symptoms can certainly give rise to emotional distress, but it's also possible to experience emotional distress—even very intense emotional distress—outside the context of mental illness. Emotional distress in this model therefore encompasses all forms of uncomfortable or aversive internal states without specifying the type or nature of this discomfort or requiring the discomfort to occur within the context of a mental illness.

My selection of decision-making style may not be as obvious, however, so we'll discuss this control parameter in detail in the next chapter. For the purposes of the present discussion, we can think about decision-making in terms of riskiness, which generally refers to the degree to which the potential costs and benefits of a decision are weighed and considered relative to each other. Decisions that disregard long-term costs and benefits while emphasizing short-term benefits may be considered "riskier," whereas decisions that emphasize long-term costs and benefits over short-term benefits may be considered "safer." I readily admit that this is a gross oversimplification of decision-making processes, but for our current purposes it's good enough.

Figure 4.4 is oriented such that moving from left to right across the control surface reflects an increase in the severity or intensity of emotional distress, whereas moving from the back to the front of the control surface reflects an increase in risky decision-making. These movements across the control surface are mirrored by corresponding movements on the behavior surface above. A left-to-right movement on the control surface, reflecting increasing emotional distress, therefore corresponds to an uphill climb on the behavior surface. An uphill climb on the behavior surface also corresponds to increasing suicide risk. A back-to-front movement on the control surface, by contrast, reflects increasingly risky decision-making but does not always correspond to an uphill climb, reflecting little to no change in suicide risk. In this model, therefore, riskier decision-making has little to no impact on suicide risk under most circumstances, with the exception of the double-folded section of the behavior surface. In this area, riskier decision-making corresponds to a very sudden uphill climb, corresponding with a rapid rise in suicide risk.

If we wanted to know the level of suicide risk that corresponds to each combination of the control parameters, we would simply go to the point on the behavior surface that was directly above that same point on the control surface. Lower levels of emotional distress and safer decision-making, for example, would be located in the upper left region of the control surface. Directly above this region of the control surface, the corresponding region of the behavior surface is located at the bottom of the hill, indicating low suicide risk. Higher levels of emotional distress and riskier decision-making, by contrast, would be located in the lower right region of the control surface. The region of the control surface directly above this area includes the plateau at the highest point of the behavior surface, indicating high suicide risk and, by default, a relatively high probability of making a suicide attempt.

Let's come back to the double fold—that important feature of the cusp catastrophe model that we temporarily put on hold earlier. Note that the double folded section of the behavior surface is located directly above the wedge-shaped region of overlap on the control surface. Outside this region of overlap, each point on the control surface corresponds to a single point on the behavior surface; there's a one-to-one match between each specific location below and a specific location above. This indicates there is only one possible level of suicide risk on the behavior surface for each combination of emotional distress and decision-making. Inside the region of overlap, however, each point on the control surface corresponds to *three* possible points on the behavior surface: the first possibility is the upper fold, the second possibility is the middle fold, and the third possibility is the lower fold. Individuals with combinations of emotional distress and decision-making that place them inside this region of overlap on the control surface could therefore have a low level of suicide risk (lower fold), intermediate level of suicide risk (middle fold), or high level of suicide risk (upper fold).

Because of the double fold, two individuals with identical levels of emotional distress and decision-making style could have very different levels of suicide risk: One may be in a low-risk state characterized by a low probability of making a suicide attempt while the other is in a high-risk state with a much higher probability of making a suicide attempt. Likewise, a single person could experience very different levels of suicide risk despite having identical levels of emotional distress and decision-making style at different points in time. Under some conditions, a person with a particular amount of emotional distress could be located on the lower fold and therefore have a low probability of making a suicide attempt (low-risk state), but under other conditions the same person with the same amount of emotional distress and same decision-making style could be located on the upper fold and therefore have a high probability of making a suicide attempt (high-risk state).

The size, shape, and location of this region of overlap can differ from person to person, such that some individuals have very large regions of overlap and others have very small regions of overlap. The model in Figure 4.5, for example, has a much larger double fold and region of overlap than the model in Figure 4.4. In this model, there are many more possible combinations of emotional distress and decision-making that could result in both high- and low-risk states. Under these circumstances, Person A could be in a high-risk state despite having a lower level of emotional distress than Person B, who could be in a low-risk state despite having a higher level of emotional distress than Person A.

The three-dimensional cusp catastrophe model also provides a practical framework for understanding how suicide risk *changes* over time; in other words, how a person shifts from a low-risk to high-risk state and vice versa. Here again, thinking topologically can be exceptionally helpful. If we were to place a ball on the behavior surface of the cusp catastrophe model, the ball

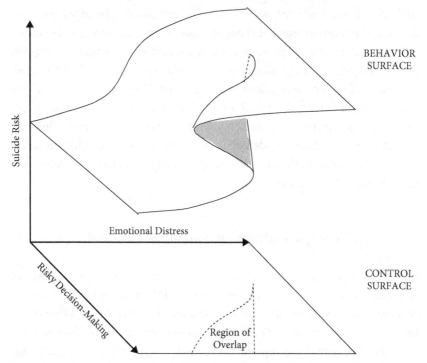

Figure 4.5 A cusp catastrophe model of suicide risk with a large region of overlap.

would naturally roll downhill, toward a lower-risk state. This would happen no matter where we place the ball on the behavior surface because gravity is a constant force that pulls the ball downhill with the same strength everywhere. Because of this constant downward force, if we were to kick the ball uphill, the ball would roll up the behavior surface's slope, gradually slow down and stop, then reverse direction and roll back downhill.

Suicide risk works the same way. When we experience something stressful in life, our emotional distress increases. Although minor and benign stressors do not cause us much emotional distress, major disruptions in life such as relationship problems or financial strain can lead to very severe emotional distress. Minor stressors are like soft or gentle kicks, whereas major stressors are like strong kicks. Major stressors cause the suicide-risk ball to travel farther up the behavior surface than minor stressors because they have more force behind them. Eventually the ball will slow down and reverse direction, however, returning to the bottom of the hill. In like fashion, acute suicidal episodes, which often occur within the context of intense emotional distress, eventually resolve as well, typically within a few minutes or hours. This natural decline in suicide risk occurs even for individuals who experience frequent and persistent suicidal thoughts and/or have made multiple suicide attempts. This topological perspective provides a way of understanding the rise and fall of suicide risk over time, as observed in Kleiman's EMA studies, our study of weekly fluctuations in suicidal thinking, and our study of social media posts. It also provides a way of understanding why some people experience slower, more gradual changes in suicide risk, whereas others experience very rapid and sudden changes; namely, that depending on where someone is located on the behavior surface, change in suicide risk can sometimes be fast and sometimes slow.

Multiple Pathways to Suicide Are Possible

I noted previously that the behavior surface of the cusp catastrophe model generally slopes upward as we move from the left to the right of the model, reflecting increasing suicide risk associated with increasing emotional distress. In contrast, suicide risk generally does not change as decision-making style changes, with the exception of the double-fold region. Along the edge of this double fold, suicide risk increases very rapidly as decision-making becomes riskier because the overlapping folds result in the coexistence of multiple possible suicide-risk states: one that is low risk (the lower fold), one that is moderate risk (the middle fold), and one that is high risk (the upper fold). This is where things get really interesting: In the cusp catastrophe model, only the lower fold and the upper fold are probable; the middle fold, by contrast, is very improbable. This means that even though all three possible states exist in this region, we will very rarely observe (or experience) the intermediate state. Because of this, when an individual moves through this particular section of the behavior surface, they could possibly "jump" suddenly from the lower fold to the upper fold—or vice versa—almost as if they were teleporting from one to the other.

In Figure 4.6, for instance, we have a cusp catastrophe model with various types of suicidal thoughts and behaviors superimposed. Being nonsuicidal

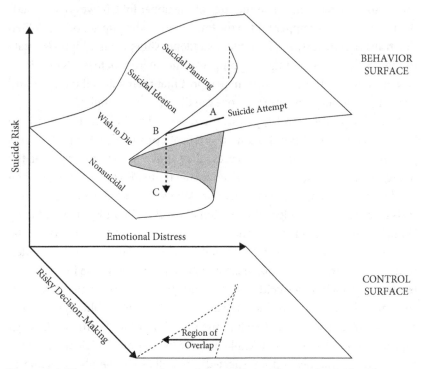

Figure 4.6 The cusp catastrophe model can account for rapid suicide risk reductions after a suicide attempt. An individual who has just made a suicide attempt begins at point A. As they experience a decline in emotional distress afterwards, they travel to the left. When they reach the edge of the upper fold of the behavior surface (point B), they suddenly "fall" to the lower fold (point C), corresponding to a rapid and sudden reduction in suicide risk.

is at the very bottom of the hill, corresponding to the lowest risk state, and as we move uphill we see various indicators of rising suicide risk: the wish to die, suicidal ideation, and suicidal planning. At the top of the behavior surface, the upper fold forms a sort of plateau that hangs over the lower fold. We see "suicide attempt" on this plateau because this is the region where the probability of making a suicide attempt is highest. Someone who has just made a suicide attempt would, therefore, be located on this region of the upper fold, perhaps at Point A. Several research studies have found that after someone has attempted suicide, they often experience a decrease in emotional distress. This reduction in emotional distress would correspond with a leftward movement along the upper fold, meaning that although the individual is experiencing a reduction in emotional distress, they are still in a high-risk state. When their level of emotional distress drops enough that the person reaches Point B on the edge of the upper fold, however, they suddenly "fall" from the upper fold to the lower fold, ending up at Point C. When this transition occurs, the individual suddenly shifts from a high-risk state to a low-risk state, seemingly skipping over the intermediate levels of suicide risk in-between. This individual may report that their suicidal thoughts and urges have significantly improved or even disappeared completely.

A similar process can happen in the reverse direction. In Figure 4.7 we have someone who is not thinking about death or suicide (Point A). As this person's emotional distress increases, they move toward the right of the figure, at which point they start experiencing thoughts about death and then maybe even some mild suicidal ideation. When their level of emotional distress reaches the right edge of the region of overlap (Point B), they suddenly "jump" from the lower fold to the upper fold, ending at Point C, where the probability of making a suicide attempt is much higher. When this sudden transition occurs, the individual effectively skips over all of the intermediate levels of risk, including suicidal ideation and planning, essentially making an "unplanned" or "impulsive" suicide attempt. The double-fold region of the cusp catastrophe model is therefore the most important feature of the cusp catastrophe model because it explains (a) why and how suicidal behaviors can emerge so rapidly and unexpectedly as well as (b) the phenomenon of nonproportionality, wherein a large increase in emotional distress can sometimes have little to no impact on suicide risk but a small increase in emotional distress can sometimes result in a very large change in suicide risk. In Figure 4.7, an initially large increase in emotional distress was associated with little change in suicide risk, but once point B was reached—the tipping point—a

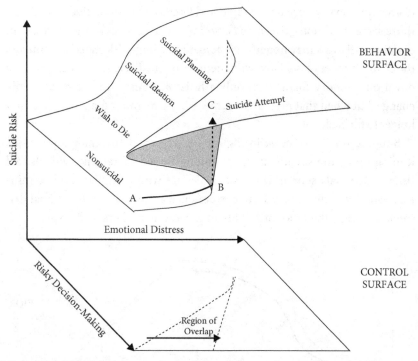

Figure 4.7 The cusp catastrophe model can account for rapid suicide risk increases prior to a suicide attempt. An individual begins in a low risk state with no thoughts of death or suicide (point A). As the experience an increase in emotional distress, they travel to the right. When they reach the edge of the lower fold of the behavior surface (point B), they suddenly "jump" to the upper fold (point C), at which point they attempt suicide.

very small incremental increase in emotional distress was associated with an enormous rise in suicide risk.

Note that, although the behavior surface is the exact same shape in Figure 4.6 and Figure 4.7, the tipping point for transitioning from a high- to low-risk state is not located in the same position as the tipping point for transitioning from a low- to high-risk state. In Figure 4.6, the tipping point for *decreasing* suicide risk corresponds to a lower level of emotional distress than the tipping point for *increasing* suicide risk. This mismatch of positions accounts for the aforementioned concept of hysteresis, which says that change in one direction does not necessarily mirror change in the opposite direction, and does not necessarily occur under the same circumstances. Under the right conditions, someone experiencing a very small increase in emotional distress may experience a very rapid and large change in suicide risk. Under those same conditions, the same person who experiences a large decrease in emotional distress may nonetheless remain in a high-risk state. This mirrors the change process associated with memory foam, discussed earlier: pressing down on memory foam, even only a little bit, causes the foam to rapidly change, but when that pressure is removed, the memory foam can take a lot longer to fill back out.

Building on these ideas, in Figure 4.8 we depict the change processes leading up to the suicide attempts among three different individuals. All three individuals start in a nonsuicidal state with a similar level of minimal emotional distress. All three experience an increase in emotional distress, although the amount of this increase differs: Person A experiences

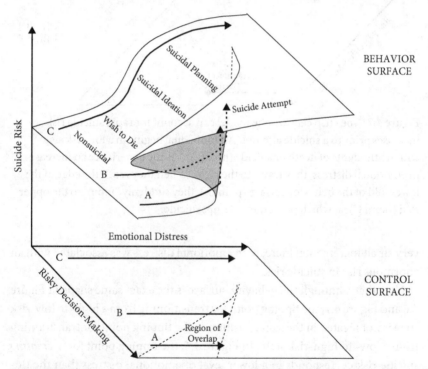

Figure 4.8 The cusp catastrophe model can account for different change processes leading up to a suicide attempt. Person A experiences a small increase in emotional distress, Person B experiences a moderate increase in emotional distress, and Person C experiences a large increase in emotional distress. All three end up in a high risk state and attempt suicide, but the level of emotional distress associated with each suicide attempt differs.

a small increase, Person B experiences a moderate increase, and Person C experiences a large increase. Despite these differences, all three transition from a low-risk state to a high-risk state, but the nature of these transitions is very different. Person A and Person B experience a catastrophic change in suicide risk when their levels of emotional distress reach the far right edge of the region of overlap, thereby passing the tipping point and jumping suddenly from the lower fold (low-risk state) to the upper fold (high-risk state). Person C, by comparison, experiences a gradual and smooth increase in suicide risk.

If we were to interview these three individuals soon after their suicide attempts, they would very likely describe different journeys. Person A would likely describe their suicide attempt as "impulsive" and would deny experiencing any suicidal thoughts or plans in the time leading up to the behavior. They would likely report a moderate level of emotional distress but probably would not meet full diagnostic criteria for a mental illness. Person B would probably describe a sequence of events beginning with the wish to die that eventually changed to suicidal ideation, but would deny suicidal planning prior to the attempt. This person also would probably score higher on various symptom checklists and questionnaires than Person A. Finally, Person C would describe experiencing the full spectrum of risk: wishing they were dead turning into suicidal ideation, after which they started thinking about how and when to attempt suicide and then, finally, putting this plan into action. They would describe a high level of emotional distress and quite likely be diagnosed with a mental illness.

The reason why all three individuals end up in a high-risk state despite experiencing different amounts of emotional distress is due to the shape of the behavior surface and, most importantly, the size and location of the double-folded region. When viewed from this perspective, we can see that many, many possible pathways to suicide can exist. Some of these pathways (Pathway C, for instance) align with our traditional assumptions about how people transition from being nonsuicidal to thinking about suicide to attempting suicide, but other pathways (Pathway A, in particular) don't fit as easily into our traditional models. The cusp catastrophe model of suicide therefore provides a useful basis for understanding how so many individuals who have attempted suicide can do so without spending much time thinking about or planning the act, and how so many suicide loss survivors can say that "everything seemed fine" in the weeks, days, and hours leading up to someone's suicide death. The cusp catastrophe model also provides a way of understanding how that Marine I met with in Iraq could have made a nearly lethal suicide attempt seemingly out of the blue.

The cusp catastrophe model also aligns with our perspective of suicide as a wicked problem. Wicked problems do not have a single right or correct solution, but rather multiple solutions that may, under certain circumstances, be better or worse than other solutions. The cusp catastrophe model of suicide shows us that there are so many possible pathways to suicide that no single strategy will be enough to sufficiently solve the problem; instead, we will need to employ multiple strategies that work under different conditions. Understanding how and why the decision to attempt suicide occurs when in a high-risk state—or, perhaps more usefully, how and why someone chooses *not* to attempt suicide when in a high-risk state—therefore warrants some consideration.

5

Marshmallows and Braking Systems

The mental illness model of suicide that has dominated the last several decades of thinking about suicide and suicide research is, historically speaking, a fairly recent development. If you're inclined to delve into the history of suicide, so to speak, there's no better source than Margaret (Peggy) Battin's book, *The Ethics of Suicide: Historical Sources*. In this book, Battin pulls together an impressive collection of writings spanning more than 4,000 years from an incredibly diverse range of cultures, nations, and faith traditions. Reviewing this compendium of work,[1] one can see that prior to the 20th century thinking about suicide was dominated by theologians, philosophers, and ethicists. Although psychological processes are frequently seen in these historical works, the mental illness model did not emerge as a prominent perspective until the 1950s, when contemporary scientific methods started to be applied systematically to understand the issue. Since the 1950s, the number of published research studies focused on suicidal thoughts and behaviors has rapidly increased. In Franklin's meta-analysis, for instance, only 3% of the 365 analyzed studies were published before 1985 and over 60% were published after 2005. The large majority of these studies (70%) involved variables and topics directly related to mental illness: internalizing disorders (e.g., anxiety, depression, hopelessness), externalizing disorders (e.g., aggression, substance use), previous suicidal thoughts and behaviors, and social factors (e.g., abuse history, stressful life events, isolation). The scientific study of suicide, which is still in its infancy, relatively speaking, is therefore heavily skewed toward the mental illness perspective.

In this chapter, we will talk about how newer theories of suicide do not meaningfully differ from conventional models of suicide and, as a result, have not advanced or changed our general thinking about or approach to suicide prevention. We will then discuss how suicide may be more usefully understood as the outcome of various decision-making processes that are influenced and shaped by a person's history and environment.

Limitations of the Mental Illness Perspective

The reason our understanding of suicide has become so strongly influenced by the mental illness model is primarily because the researchers who have conducted the bulk of suicide-focused studies in the past few decades hail from the mental health disciplines, especially clinical psychology and psychiatry. Consistent with the recent zeitgeist, some of the newer and most popular theories of suicide introduced within the past decades have also come from mental health professionals and have tended to emphasize psychological processes. The interpersonal-psychological theory of suicide, for instance, argues that suicide results from the combination of perceived burdensomeness (the belief that one is a liability on others), thwarted belongingness (the perception that one is isolated and disconnected from others), and capability for suicide (the ability to endure physical and psychological pain). Similarly, the three-step theory of suicide argues that suicide occurs when psychological pain—which could include various sources and types of emotional distress—exceeds one's connectedness with others and when the individual possesses the capability for suicide. Meanwhile, the integrated motivational volitional theory of suicide incorporates many of these same variables and constructs, but emphasizes two other psychological concepts: defeat (the belief that one is a failure and humiliated) and entrapment (the perception that one has no available solutions).

Unfortunately, these newer theories have not performed much better than the old. Across more than two dozen research studies, for instance, Carol Chu and colleagues found that the average correlations of perceived burdensomeness, thwarted belongingness, and capability for suicide with suicide attempts never exceeded $r = 0.25$, which is approximately equal to an odds ratio of 2.6, similar to findings. This is only slightly larger in size than the average odds ratios among various types of mental illness and suicide attempts discussed previously in Chapter 2, which range from 1.3 to 2.1. Prominent risk factors and concepts from newer theories of suicide do not appear to explain suicide much better than more general theories that emphasize mental illness, though, mostly because the concepts proposed by these newer theories are not all that different from mental illness in general. Feeling that people would be better off without you (i.e., burdensomeness), for example, is not all that different from feelings of worthlessness—one of nine symptoms of a major depressive episode.

Likewise, feeling like a failure (i.e., defeat) and that one has no available solutions (i.e., entrapment) is not all that different from the fixation on past failures and hopelessness that are also listed as symptoms of major depressive disorder. Because of this, the concepts proposed by newer suicide theories cannot be meaningfully distinguished from mental illness more generally.

This is probably why reductions in theory-specific concepts do not explain reductions in suicide attempts among the handful of treatments that have been shown to prevent suicide attempts. In 2018, I published the results of a study designed to determine if reductions in the concepts specific to the interpersonal psychological theory of suicide (burdensomeness, belonging, and capability for suicide) differed between a treatment that reduces suicide attempts and another treatment that was less effective for preventing suicide attempts. In that study, my hope was that we would begin to figure out why some treatments were better at stopping people from trying to kill themselves. What was actually changing in people who received these treatments? If we could figure out what these treatments were changing, and could link those changes to reductions in suicide attempts, we might be able to improve existing treatments and also develop new strategies that could change the things that mattered the most.

Our results from that study showed that patients in both treatments reported similar improvements in burdensomeness, belonging, and capability for suicide. Both treatments were therefore pretty good at reducing some things believed to cause suicide, but one of the two treatments was much better at preventing suicide attempts. This pattern suggests the better treatment must have been stopping people from killing themselves because it was changing something other than burdensomeness, belonging, and capability for suicide. Interestingly, we had previously found this same pattern when we looked at how these treatments improved depression and anxiety symptoms. Treatment studies conducted by other researchers have found similar patterns. Overall, these studies suggest that the central concepts described by many of the newer theories were not all that different from other, more general indicators of mental illness. The reasons why some treatments and interventions are better at preventing suicide attempts therefore remain unknown, but there is now a fair amount of evidence that the reasons probably involve something other than mental illness.

A Different Perspective

In our efforts to test and improve treatments and interventions for suicide prevention, we have routinely asked patients to tell us what they found to be most helpful and unhelpful about the treatments they had received. We also asked for them to tell us about times when they were in crisis but did *not* attempt suicide. What did you do to keep yourself from attempting suicide? How were you able to handle that situation? What did you do differently this time? What was most helpful to you during that crisis? We asked these particular questions because, as treatment researchers, we were interested more in what contributed to the *prevention* or avoidance of suicidal behaviors than in what contributed to the *emergence* of suicidal behaviors. In other words, we didn't just ask people to tell us why they attempted suicide; we also asked them why they did *not* attempt suicide even when they had a very strong desire or urge to do so. These two questions may sound like splitting hairs, but they're not; because of hysteresis, the fifth assumption of emergence, change in one direction is not necessarily the same as change in the opposite direction. As applied to suicide, the processes that propel someone toward suicide may be different from the processes that stop this forward momentum and/ or move someone away from suicide.

To understand how this works, imagine yourself driving a car. If you want to go faster, you push down on the accelerator, thereby activating a chain of events that cause your vehicle to speed up. If you want to slow down, you can remove your foot from the accelerator, but if you want to slow down very fast and stop, then you can also push down on the brake, thereby activating a *different* chain of events that decelerates the vehicle. Pushing down on the accelerator and pushing down on the brake involve completely different components of the car that work in very different ways. Pushing the accelerator down will cause the car to go faster, but removing your foot from the accelerator or even pulling the accelerator pedal up will only slow you down a little bit. Pushing the brake, however, will cause the car to slow down a lot, but removing your foot from the brake or pulling up on the brake pedal will not increase the car's speed by much.

According to our patients, this was a useful way of thinking about things. Our patients still encountered highly distressing situations during which they typically experienced extreme emotional activation. This felt like pushing down on the accelerator, propelling themselves towards suicide. Because of the treatment, however, they were learning to make different decisions in response to these situations. Specifically, they were choosing to use the brake, slowing themselves down and stopping themselves before they collided with suicide. In many ways, this wasn't surprising to us because the treatments we were developing weren't designed to *completely* eliminate stress and problems in life; they were designed to help people respond differently and more effectively to these types of situations. Patients confirmed that this is exactly what was happening; when they were heading toward a collision in the midst of a highly stressful situation with an unknown outcome, instead of simply lifting their foot off the accelerator and hoping for the best, they started to apply pressure to the brake instead, thereby avoiding the collision in most circumstances. "I never know what's going to happen in the end," one patient explained to me, "but I've learned it's in my best interest to just slow down for a bit to see how things play out before making any decisions." Another patient described this process in a somewhat different way: "It's sort of like that marshmallow experiment; just because I *want* to act upon an urge doesn't mean I *have* to."

The marshmallow experiment

The "marshmallow experiment" is a famous series of research studies that examined decision-making processes among children. The basic concept of the study involved presenting a single marshmallow to a child along with a choice: the child could either eat the marshmallow now or, if he waited a short period of time (typically around 15 minutes) without eating the marshmallow, he could receive a second marshmallow. The marshmallow experiment was not a single study, as implied by its name, but rather a series of studies conducted by psychologist Walter Mischel at Stanford University in the 1960s and 1970s. A central feature of these studies was the use of marshmallows as a desirable reward, although cookies and pretzels were sometimes used as rewards instead. It was the marshmallow, though, that ultimately became the studies' namesake. No matter which treat was used, the central purpose of these studies was to understand the principles involved in delayed gratification, the process by which we resist the temptation of a reward that is immediately available in order to obtain a larger reward that will only become available at a later time.

Various iterations of this concept were subsequently tested to examine various factors that might influence a child's ability to delay gratification. For example, in one study children were presented with the marshmallow choice after participating in activities designed to lead them to view the researcher as either trustworthy or untrustworthy. This enabled the researchers to examine how different levels of perceived trust impacted decision-making. Not surprisingly, results of this particular study suggested children were less willing to wait for the second marshmallow if they received instructions from an untrustworthy source. Most of us can relate; what if an untrustworthy source promises us that a bigger reward is forthcoming only if we turn down the smaller reward that is immediately available? What if they're lying and a bigger reward isn't coming after all? If true, we could miss out on the small reward available now. Under these conditions, it's understandable that we are less likely to wait for that second marshmallow and will instead take what we can get now.

In another iteration of the experiment, researchers manipulated whether or not the marshmallow remained in sight while the children waited. This enabled researchers to examine whether decision-making differs when the reward is constantly in our faces (and within reach) as opposed to when the reward is out of sight and not immediately attainable. Here again, the results probably aren't surprising: we're less likely to wait for a bigger reward when we can see the smaller reward and easily grab it. It's much easier to wait, however, when we can't see that smaller reward. Out of sight, out of mind. Other manipulations to this basic paradigm were tested, all of them being designed to understand how the decisions a child makes with respect to short- versus long-term rewards are influenced by the situation. Some children may, for instance, be reasonably good at delaying gratification in some situations, but under other circumstances they may not be willing or able to delay gratification at all. Similarly, some children may struggle to delay gratification in some situations, but under different circumstances they may be willing and able to do it after all. Decision-making is therefore influenced by the context within which the decision has to be made. Will a child choose one marshmallow now or wait for a second marshmallow? Well, it depends.

Several years after conducting his studies, Mischel followed up with some of the children who participated in the original studies and found that those who were able to wait longer for their rewards as a child scored much higher during their teenage years on standardized academic testing and were more likely to receive high ratings on various questionnaires and measures of self-control and ability to handle stress. Now teenagers, these children were also more likely to stay focused during various tasks. Several decades later—40 years after the original studies were conducted—some of the children, now adults, were tracked down yet again and asked to participate in a number of additional research studies. These latter studies found that individuals who were better able to delay gratification as children showed greater levels of self-control as adults. Those with greater levels of self-control also demonstrated higher levels of brain activity in the prefrontal cortex, a region of the brain involved in decision-making processes, reducing emotional distress, and inhibiting or controlling one's actions. In contrast, brain activity in the ventral striatum, a region of the brain involved in processing the value of desires and rewards, was reduced. The overall conclusion of Mischel's many studies was that delayed gratification in childhood predicted greater brain activity and performance on several metrics of self-control, academic performance, and stress management measured many, many years later. These latter findings understandably catapulted the marshmallow experiment to fame.

Not everyone shared the excitement, however. Some researchers questioned the conclusions, noting that they did not take into account a number of important limitations in the original studies that could have influenced the results. For example, the children who participated in these studies were enrolled at Stanford University's on-campus preschool, meaning they came from a community that did not necessarily represent the broader spectrum of U.S. children. If the marshmallow experiment were conducted with children representing a wider and more diverse range of communities, would the same patterns be observed? Researchers also noted that only one in four of the children who originally participated in a marshmallow experiment study could be contacted for the follow-up studies conducted years later during adolescence. The long-term results reported by Mischel were therefore based on only a small subset of all the children who participated. This subset of children who were willing to participate many years later may have differed in a number of ways from those who could not be contacted or were unwilling to participate again. It's also entirely possible that the families who were contacted and the families who were not contacted actually are similar to one another, in which case the results and conclusions are likely to be valid after all. Unfortunately, we simply cannot know. Drawing conclusions about *everyone* based on only a small subset of the original participants is risky and potentially error-prone.

In light of these (and other) concerns, a team of researchers led by Tyler Watts attempted to replicate the marshmallow experiment in a study that was designed to address many of these limitations. Their results, published in 2018, were similar to those of Mischel's original studies, although the correlations were much smaller. Their findings also suggested that environmental and contextual factors (e.g., parental education level, availability of toys and books in the home, parental use of physical punishment) play a really important role that should not be ignored. Some have interpreted these latter findings as "debunking" the original conclusions of the marshmallow experiment studies and have concluded instead that the ability to delay gratification has nothing (or perhaps very little) to do at all with any of the desirable outcomes originally described by Mischel. I would argue, however, that this is a flawed interpretation of the data, because this finding still aligns with Mischel's central conclusion regarding decision-making processes: context matters.

In Watts's replication study, delayed gratification differed among children who lived in homes and communities with divergent levels of economic and social advantage. One possible reason for this is that children raised in disadvantaged homes and communities are more likely to have lives characterized by uncertainty. For example, parents who earn a lower income may be unable to follow through with a promised reward due to financial hardship. Under these circumstances, children may learn that a reward available now may not always be available later. The decision to delay gratification (or not) is therefore intertwined with environmental context, such that decision-making cannot be meaningfully separated from the circumstances within which the choice is presented. The same is true for suicide: We cannot meaningfully separate the decision to make a suicide attempt from the circumstances within which the choice is presented.

The influence of context was the key idea that motivated Mischel to conduct the marshmallow experiment in the first place. Mischel believed that attempts to understand and predict human behavior based on combinations of various personality "traits" was inadequate and fundamentally flawed. He also believed that behavior occurred as a consequence of conditional thinking, such that people make decisions about acting (or not acting) based upon what was happening to them and around them on a moment-to-moment basis. The decisions we make do not reflect who we are so much as they reflect what is happening to us. Personality and psychological traits are widely presumed to be a primary driver of human behavior, mostly because they are presumed to be relatively fixed or constant over time and situations. In reality, however, personality and psychological traits are notoriously unreliable as predictors of human behavior because individuals often make different decisions and/or engage in different behaviors under different conditions. When the conditions that surround us change, our decisions and behaviors can change as well. For example, those who are shy or uncomfortable in large groups of strangers may be talkative and relaxed in smaller groups of close friends. Likewise, a person who is boisterous and obnoxious in the workplace may be quiet and restrained when being disciplined by a supervisor.

Mental illness and its symptoms tend to behave in a similar way; neither fixed nor constant, they change over time, often in response to the environment. Symptoms can be very pronounced and severe in some circumstances but minimal or hardly noticeable in other circumstances. Behavior, whether choosing to eat (or not eat) a marshmallow or making (or not making) a suicide attempt, therefore results from an ever-changing decision-making process that occurs within the context of ever-changing environments. From this perspective, mental illness and emotional distress more generally is better understood as one particular context within which the decision to make a suicide attempt or not often presents itself. This does not mean, however, that mental illness is the *only* context within which this choice is considered. This also does not mean that mental illness *causes* suicide, just as leaving a marshmallow within eyesight of a hungry child does not cause the child to eat it. These conditions certainly influence the probability of one choice being made over another, but many other conditions and factors influence these decisions as well. This gets at the heart of what the aforementioned patient was describing when she said that she didn't have to act upon every suicidal urge: she came to realize that she could choose to act or choose *not* to act even in highly distressing situations, where the perceived value of suicide is magnified.

A marshmallow test for adults

The basic concept involved in the marshmallow experiment—decision-making under different conditions—has received increased attention in the past decade among suicide researchers, although not nearly enough attention, in my opinion. Researchers working with suicidal adults usually don't offer marshmallows as the reward to be chosen, although I recognize that some of us adults might find eating a marshmallow or two (or three or four) highly rewarding. Researchers typically offer another reward instead: money. Consider, for example, some of the decision-making research conducted by Alexandre Dombrovski. One of the methods Dombrovski has used in his research is called the Monetary Choice Questionnaire (MCQ). In the MCQ, individuals are asked multiple times if they would prefer to receive a smaller amount of money now or receive another, larger amount of money later. With each choice, three conditions are changed: the amount of the smaller reward that could be received now, the amount of the larger reward that could be received later, and the amount of time that must pass before the larger reward can be received. For example, a research participant might be asked to choose their preferred option in each of the three following scenarios:

$5 now or $6 in one week;
$5 now or $75 in one month; and
$50 now or $75 in two weeks.

What would you pick in these three different scenarios? For the first scenario, you might prefer to receive $5 now because neither $5 nor $6 is a particularly large sum of money and waiting an entire week to receive only one extra dollar may not seem to be worth it. For the second scenario, however, you might prefer to wait an entire month to receive $75 because this amount is a lot larger than $5. If you chose to take $5 now in the first scenario but in the second scenario chose to decline $5 now and wait instead, it's probably because the perceived value of $5 in the second scenario seems much less than the perceived value of $5 in the first scenario. It's the same dollar amount but this time around, the larger amount that you have to wait for makes the $5 seem much less valuable, so waiting is worth it. For the third scenario, the decision might not be as straightforward as the first two, however. In this scenario, you might consider $75 to be a meaningful and worthwhile increase in value over $50, but you might be ambivalent about whether or not the extra $25 is worth waiting two weeks. How you ultimately decide to weigh this increase in monetary value relative to the length of wait will probably be influenced to some degree by your life circumstances. If you are experiencing financial strain and have an unpaid bill due within the next few days, you may prefer to take $50 now, even though you would typically choose to wait for the bigger amount. If you are not financially strained, however, waiting a few weeks for the extra amount may work out better for you. Context matters.

The MCQ uses a scoring algorithm that takes into account the difference between the values of each option (this is called the *reward discount*) as well as the length of the time between each option (this is called the *delay*). By combining these two factors across multiple choices, the MCQ provides an overall score called the *delayed reward discount*. Dombrovski used the MCQ to examine how individuals who have thought about and/or attempted suicide tend to make decisions as compared to individuals who had never attempted suicide, and he found a number of patterns:

1. People who were thinking about suicide were less likely to wait for the larger monetary amount than those who were not suicidal;
2. People who had made a low-lethality suicide attempt (i.e., a suicide attempt that was unlikely to result in death) were less likely to wait for the larger monetary amount than those who were not suicidal;
3. People who had made a high-lethality suicide attempt (i.e., a suicide attempt that was nearly fatal) were more likely to wait for the larger monetary amount than those who were thinking about suicide and those who had made a low-lethality suicide attempt; and
4. People who had made a high-lethality suicide attempt were no different from those who were nonsuicidal.

These results suggest that, when weighing the pros and cons of acting now versus acting later, individuals who have thought about suicide and made low-lethality suicide attempts in the past are less likely to wait for a bigger reward; they prefer the smaller reward available now. Individuals who had never attempted suicide and individuals who had made nearly lethal suicide attempts in the past, by contrast, were more likely to wait for the bigger reward.

I want to emphasize this latter finding: the decision-making process of someone who almost died as a result of their suicide attempt was no different from the decision-making process of someone who had never attempted suicide, was not currently suicidal, and did not have a mental illness. This is an especially important finding because it shows us that some who engage in suicidal behaviors have a decision-making style that is no different from those who do not have a mental illness and have never tried to kill themselves. This finding lines up with the idea that there can be multiple pathways to suicide: Some involve a preference for eating the one marshmallow available now instead of waiting for a second, but others involve a preference for waiting for two marshmallows instead of eating the one that's available right now.

Balancing potential gains with potential losses

Let's consider another research study that used the Iowa Gambling Task, a different method for understanding decision-making styles. The Iowa Gambling Task is a game-like procedure that involves choosing a card from one of four separate decks of cards. When you choose a card, you either win money or you simultaneously win *and* lose money. The four decks of cards differ from one another with respect to the probability and magnitude of these two possible outcomes, such that some decks are more likely to result in winning money, whereas other decks are more likely to result in losing money. Critically, the decks that are most helpful for winning the game have a greater number of cards that combine small wins with smaller losses (e.g., win $5 but lose $3), resulting in a net gain over time, albeit a slow and gradual gain. Conversely, the decks that are least helpful have more cards that provide large wins combined with larger losses (e.g., win $1,000 but lose $1,100), resulting in a net loss over time. At its core, the Iowa Gambling Task assesses one's willingness to develop and employ an effective long-term strategy for reward at the expense of satisfying a short-term desire for a much bigger, but potentially more costly, reward. Because you don't know when you will get winning cards or losing cards, a "slow and steady" decision-making style ultimately provides the best strategy for winning the Iowa Gambling Task.

Fabrice Jollant used the Iowa Gambling Task to understand how slow and steady versus risky decision-making style was associated with suicidal behavior, and found that people who had used a violent method for making a suicide attempt (e.g., using a firearm, or trying to strangulate themselves) were associated with increased use of a risky decision-making style. In uncertain situations, those who used highly dangerous methods for attempting suicide therefore showed a preference for "big gains" even though the pursuit of these gains typically resulted in even bigger losses. When we consider the results of Jollant's research in combination with Dombrovski's research, they together suggest that people who use more violent methods to attempt suicide have a preference for big rewards. The contexts within which these preferences were pursued, however, differed across the two studies. In Dombrovski's study, the bigger reward was available under conditions of certainty: Before making a decision, you know how long you have to wait to get the bigger reward and also know how much bigger the reward will be if you wait. In Jollant's study, by comparison, the bigger reward was available under conditions of *un*certainty: you might win big, or you might lose big—but the outcome couldn't be known in advance. In Dombrovski's study, the preference for a bigger reward generally worked in the person's favor: In the end, the preference for big rewards resulted in a bigger sum of money received. In Jollant's study, the preference for a bigger reward worked against the person, resulting in a big loss. Preference for bigger rewards, therefore, isn't right or wrong. Sometimes it is better than a preference for smaller rewards, and other times it is worse.

Jollant also has conducted research seeking to uncover whether an individual's understanding of the available choices makes any difference. Using the Iowa Gambling Task again, Jollant found that those with a mental illness or a previous suicide attempt were less likely to understand how a "winning" strategy in the Iowa Gambling Task could lead to better outcomes. In the Iowa Gambling Task, a winning strategy involves adopting a slow and steady approach that results in smaller wins that, over time, accumulate. Those with a mental illness who were able to articulate this strategy were able to put the strategy into action. As a result, they won more money than people with a mental illness who could not figure out this strategy. Individuals with a prior suicide attempt were just as likely to understand the winning strategy and how it worked, but this understanding was *not* correlated with positive outcomes because they did not actually use this strategy. Individuals with a mental illness benefited therefore from knowing how to win the game, but individuals who had attempted suicide didn't use the winning strategy even when they knew that it would work. Why wouldn't someone use a strategy that they know works?

Making choices in uncertain situations

One possible answer to this question may come from yet another study conducted by Dombrovski, which investigated a different aspect of decision-making called *probabilistic reversal learning*. Probabilistic reversal learning involves the capacity to learn a particular rule for making correct decisions to obtain a desired result and then learning a different rule for making correct decisions to obtain that same result when the original rule no longer works. To examine how this was related to suicidal thoughts and behaviors, Dombrovski presented subjects with pairs of cards and asked them to pick the correct card but didn't tell them what it was that made a card correct or incorrect. Each card had a different number of shapes that varied in color. For example, one card might have three blue squares and the second card might have five red circles. To win, you had to figure out which property of the card was correct (e.g., a particular color, a particular shape, a particular number of items). If the rule is "blue," for example, you only win if you select the cards with blue shapes. If the rule is "three," however, you win only if you select the cards with three shapes. This is the "learning" part of the task. When you choose the correct card, you receive a reward most (but not all) of the time, and when you choose the incorrect card, you receive a punishment most (but not all) of the time. This is the "probabilistic" part of the task: Making a correct decision does not guarantee you always will be rewarded, and making an incorrect decision does not guarantee you always will be punished.

At a certain point during the game, the winning rule unexpectedly changes, such that your previously successful decision-making style results in punishment more often than reward. Critically, no one tells you that the rule has changed; you have to figure that out on your own. If the rule was originally "blue," for instance, and you select this option again after the rule changes to "circles," you will be punished instead of rewarded. This is the "reversal" part of the task. This rule reversal enables us to determine if individuals are able to (a) quickly identify and learn a successful decision-making strategy that leads to success under conditions of uncertainty, (b) preserve a successful strategy even when occasionally obtaining an undesired result, (c) quickly adapt to an unexpected change in circumstances, and (d) preserve a newly learned decision-making strategy even when occasionally obtaining an undesired result.

Probabilistic reversal learning involves a lot of different concepts, but they serve as really good models for life. Sometimes when we make decisions that have worked well for us in the past, we nonetheless experience an undesired outcome, and sometimes when we make "bad" decisions we nonetheless experience success. We often call this bad luck and good luck. Sometimes the circumstances of life change unexpectedly, though, such that the decisions that were useful to us in the past no longer work. When this happens, we can either stick to what worked in the past, even though it's no longer working now, or we can adapt and figure out a new strategy that works better under these new conditions. Even when we figure out a new effective strategy, though, it won't lead to desired outcomes all the time. Here again, we can't escape luck; sometimes making the right decision leads to a bad outcome anyway, through no fault of our own (bad luck), and sometimes making the wrong decision nonetheless leads to a good outcome (good luck). At this point, we can either stick with the new strategy that works most of the time or we can abandon this strategy to seek out yet another strategy. Unfortunately, switching strategies in response to bad luck actually *decreases* our chances of success because we effectively have moved away from something that works most of the time.

Dombrovski's results suggest this is where individuals who have attempted suicide struggle the most: They tend to abandon too quickly newly learned and largely successful, though not perfect, strategies. As a result, they experience punishment more often than success. Under these circumstances, it's easy to see how depression, hopelessness, and a sense of entrapment and despair can arise and persist over time. This brings us to another question: Why don't individuals who have made a suicide attempt use strategies that they know will work better? Well, one possible reason is that we sometimes pay more attention to the times when a strategy did *not* work, even though these instances are rare and uncommon. If we place too much weight on the times that a strategy did *not* work, we are more likely to stop using strategies that work most of the time.

This is something I've heard from many suicidal people, especially the patients I've treated over the years. They have, for example, explained that they stopped calling a friend because the friend was unhelpful or unavailable once in a time of need. Never mind that the friend was there all the other times they needed help—that one time was enough to abandon this strategy. I've also heard many of my patients talk about how they've stopped doing things such as going to the gym because a staff member there was rude the last time they went; or they've stopped engaging in a hobby because they still felt stressed or unhappy afterward, so they decided that it didn't work. When experiencing intense distress and faced with uncertainty, we must develop the ability to shift our attention away from the times that something *didn't* work as desired and make sure that we pay attention to the times that same thing *did* work. Just because something doesn't work all the time doesn't mean it'll never work.

An Internal Braking System

The ability to inhibit a behavior—to resist an action we feel compelled to pursue—is associated with certain patterns of activity in our brains. Walter Mischel's follow-up research with the marshmallow experiment participants, conducted several decades after these children were first presented with the choice between eating a single marshmallow or waiting for two, found different patterns of activation in the prefrontal cortex and ventral striatum among those who had waited as compared to those who had not. Those who had, as children, waited for the second marshmallow tended to have increased activity in the prefrontal cortex and decreased activity in the ventral striatum. The prefrontal cortex is located at the very front of the brain, right behind our forehead, and is involved in how we organize our thoughts and behaviors in ways that help us to achieve our goals. The ventral striatum is located in the center of the brain and is involved in the anticipation of future rewards, the perception and experience of reward, and learning from prior experience. In combination, these two regions of the brain are critical for decision-making, especially decisions that involve the inhibition or stopping of actions that are inconsistent with our desired goals and intentions. We have our prefrontal cortex and the ventral striatum to thank when we get angry but choose not to become violent or aggressive, when we feel overwhelmed by stress but then put together a plan to resolve the situation, and when we're upset and want to do something destructive but decide against it. Together, these regions of the brain function as an internal braking system.

Under ideal conditions, these two brain structures work together in a co-ordinated manner. When we are confronted with an uncertain and stressful situation, our ventral striatum provides information about options that may lead to successful or desired outcomes, and our prefrontal cortex weighs the pros and cons of these various options. When we think about an option that we expect to be successful, our ventral striatum activates. So does one particular region of our prefrontal cortex called the ventromedial prefrontal cortex. When we think about an option that is unlikely to be successful, however, the ventral striatum and ventromedial prefrontal cortex do not activate. Many individuals who have attempted suicide do not show these patterns of activation. When they are thinking about potentially successful options, their ventral striatum and ventromedial prefrontal cortex do not activate as much as these regions do among individuals who have not attempted suicide. As a result, options that are more likely to succeed do not carry much more perceived value than options that are less likely to succeed. "Obvious" strategies and solutions, therefore, may not be so obvious to someone who is vulnerable to making a suicide attempt.

This problem can be magnified when someone is highly distressed. This is because the ventromedial prefrontal cortex also seems to be involved in processing emotions, both positive and negative. Among those who have attempted suicide, the part of the ventromedial prefrontal cortex that processes negative emotions such as anxiety, fear, and disgust tends to become overactivated when in stressful situations, especially stressful or uncomfortable interpersonal situations. At the same time, the part of the ventromedial prefrontal cortex that processes positive emotions such as joy, hope, and contentment tends to be underactivated. Because positive emotions and expectations serve to modulate or counteract the effects of negative emotions and expectations, the combination of overactivity in certain areas of the brain and underactivity in other areas can result in heightened sensitivity to stressful situations and increased emotional distress, especially situations with uncertain outcomes. In the presence of such intense, unmodulated emotional distress with no expectation of success or positive outcome, risky "all-in" or "Hail Mary" decisions become more probable.

Being able to anticipate the consequences of our decisions and actions—both good and bad—helps us to weigh the options available to us and, critically, to inhibit those options that carry a high cost despite their immediate allure. If we expect good things to happen to us, we are more likely to hit the brakes; we may choose to forego the single marshmallow that's available right now because we expect that a second marshmallow will eventually become available. We also may choose to pursue a safer decision-making style that results in smaller rewards in the short-term because we realize that, over the long run, lots of little wins eventually add up. Expecting good outcomes also lends itself to preserving a successful decision-making strategy even when it fails from time to time. If, however, we have little reason to expect that our decisions will yield any reward—or if we are unable to recognize how these decisions will yield any reward—we may be less inclined to avoid making a risky, all-in decision.

In order to "win" the biggest rewards, people must therefore choose *not* to act while in the presence of a smaller reward (delayed reward discounting), choose *against* an option that promises a payoff but also a potentially bigger loss (risky decision-making), or choose *not* to abandon a decision-making strategy despite uncertainty and periodic failure (probabilistic reversal learning). Without a braking system, the probability of collision is increased. When speeding toward a collision, taking your foot off the accelerator can cause you to slow down, but this alone may not be enough to stop your forward momentum. In these circumstances, you also need good brakes.

This has major implications for suicide. Reducing emotional distress and mental illness is certainly helpful, but that strategy alone may not be enough to stop someone's forward momentum toward suicide. The ability to quickly identify and utilize self-regulatory strategies is also essential, and these concepts are central to the treatments that are most effective for reducing the occurrence of suicidal behaviors. Considerable research supports the value of these approaches, but mental health professionals rarely use them when working with suicidal or high-risk patients. In the next chapter we will look at why this may be.

6

Handwashing and Changing
the Status Quo

Up until 19th century, women who were giving birth typically delivered their babies at home, assisted by female relatives, friends, and a midwife. Childbirth was a dangerous and potentially life-threatening event for both the mother and the baby. With each additional pregnancy, the dice were rolled again. Because of this risk, upper class women started requesting physician-assisted childbirths beginning in the middle 18th century, a cultural shift prompted in large part by the rapid scientific advances in biology and chemistry that introduced an array of new medical treatments and procedures, such as anesthesia, surgical techniques, and medications. Many infections, injuries, and conditions previously assumed to be fatal were now potentially treatable and even survivable. In light of these remarkable medical advances, women hoped that physician-assisted childbirth would provide similar life-saving benefits.

At first, physicians helped to deliver babies in women's homes, consistent with tradition and historical precedent. Over time, however, more and more women decided to deliver their babies in hospitals instead. The relocation of childbirth from the home to the hospital provided some benefits for women; hemorrhaging and other medical complications, for instance, could be treated more rapidly and effectively in hospitals than homes. What no one expected, however, was how this relocation could introduce other potentially deadly risks to women, namely increased exposure to infectious diseases. Infections could happen anywhere, of course, but they were much more common for women who gave birth in hospitals as compared to women who gave birth at home. Puerperal fever, in particular, was especially common after childbirth and could be fatal. Giving birth in a hospital, where women were under the watchful eyes of physicians and other medical professionals, was supposed to be safer than giving birth at home. In many cases, however, the opposite was true: Giving birth in a hospital could *increase* a woman's risk of infection and death.

This was the unfortunate situation at the Vienna General Hospital in the mid-19th century. At that time, the hospital had two clinics for childbirth, one run by physicians (the obstetrical clinic) and one run by midwives (the midwife's ward). Ignaz Semmelweis, a Hungarian physician who worked in the hospital, noticed that the mortality rate among women who gave birth in the obstetrical clinic was approximately double the mortality rate among women who gave birth in the midwife's ward. Even more alarming, the death rate in the obstetrical clinic was actually higher than the death rate among women who gave birth *on the street outside the hospital*. Things were so bad in the obstetrical clinic that women would beg to be placed in the midwife's clinic instead, and some would even try to sneak out of the obstetrical clinic when going into labor. Confronted with this perplexing situation, Semmelweis wondered what might be contributing to this problem and how the hospital could fix it.

To answer this question, Semmelweis generated several hypotheses and subsequently tested each in a systematic manner. Some hypotheses, in retrospect and with the benefit of hindsight bias (to include somewhere around 200 additional years of knowledge), were less plausible than others. Semmelweis first observed that in the obstetrical clinic, women gave birth on their backs but in the midwife's ward, women gave birth on their sides. Semmelweis therefore had women in the obstetrical clinic give birth on their sides, but this did not change mortality rates. Semmelweis next observed that when a woman in the obstetrical clinic died of puerperal fever, priests would walk through the clinic and ring a bell; they didn't do this when a woman died in the midwife's clinic, though. He wondered if this ritual was increasing women's anxiety, thereby causing the fever. Semmelweis directed the priests to stop ringing their bells and to change their path through the clinic, but this did not reduce mortality rates either.

After more time had passed, Semmelweis observed another key difference between the two clinics: the physicians who delivered babies in the obstetrical clinic conducted autopsies on cadavers in the hospital morgue, but midwives did not perform any work in the morgue and did not have any contact with cadavers. Semmelweis additionally observed that if a physician's patient went into labor while they were conducting an autopsy, the physician often went directly from the autopsy room to the obstetrical clinic to perform the delivery. Although the physicians washed their hands before leaving the autopsy room, Semmelweis noticed that a strong odor nonetheless lingered on their hands. Based on this observation, Semmelweis speculated that tiny pieces of corpse, which he called "cadaverous particles," must remain on the physicians' hands even after they had been washed. Semmelweis further hypothesized that these cadaverous particles were the source of the odor, and that this odor was, in turn, causing puerperal fever.

The notion of infectious diseases being caused by odors may seem silly to us now, but in the 18th century this idea wasn't such a harebrained idea. Indeed, it was a generally accepted theory. These infection-causing odors were called *miasma*, a term derived from the ancient Greek word for "pollution." Semmelweis speculated that these cadaverous particles were causing miasma on physicians' hands and miasma, in turn, were being transferred to the women during childbirth and causing puerperal fever. To test this idea, Semmelweis ordered his physicians to start cleaning their hands and instruments with a chlorinated lime solution, even if they had washed their hands using some other method, because he believed chlorinated lime solution would be the most effective method for eliminating the foul miasma odor. Once this new handwashing procedure was instituted, puerperal fever and fever-related mortality rates dropped significantly in the obstetrics clinic, to a level that was comparable to the mortality rate in the midwife's ward. Introducing handwashing with chlorinated lime solution meant that women were no longer more likely to die after physician-assisted childbirth as compared to midwife-assisted childbirth.

Semmelweis's achievement is remarkable not just because he figured out how to solve a life-threatening problem; it's also remarkable because he identified a solution with almost no understanding of the underlying processes that were actually causing these deaths—germs. At that time, germ theory hadn't been invented yet. The existence of microorganisms had been hypothesized by researchers many years before, but the idea was not yet accepted by the broader scientific community because no one had yet been able to physically see these invisible entities or prove definitively that they existed. In this absence of such evidence, the notion of microorganisms was actively resisted and even rejected by leading scientists and the medical community. Semmelweis therefore figured out how to prevent a particular cause of death without knowing what its cause actually was.

Tragically, the idea that ultimately led to his unique handwashing solution stemmed from the death of someone close to him. While Semmelweis was trying to figure out the problem of puerperal fever, a pathologist friend contracted a fever and died soon thereafter. Pathologists are medical professionals who study the causes and effects of diseases by closely examining human tissue samples. During the mid-19th century, pathologists had very high mortality rates because they contracted various illnesses, infections, and diseases much more often than other medical professionals. In the absence of germ theory, no one really understood why pathologists were so susceptible to these conditions and early death. Today, however, we do: They were contracting infections and diseases from germs that were active in the tissue samples and bodies they were inspecting. When Semmelweis's friend contracted a fever and died, Semmelweis recognized that the pathologist's symptoms were consistent with puerperal fever, the very same condition that caused the deaths of so many women soon after childbirth. Prior to his friend's death, Semmelweis had only seen puerperal fever among women who had recently given birth and had mistakenly assumed—like so many other physicians of his time—that puerperal fever affected women only. When Semmelweis learned that right before falling ill his friend had conducted an autopsy on a female patient who had died of puerperal fever, he correctly deduced that the fever had probably been transferred from the female cadaver to the pathologist via physical contact.

Semmelweis was not the only person piecing this together. Other medical professionals around the world were arriving at similar conclusions based on their own observations of the benefits of handwashing with soap and other antiseptic solutions. Florence Nightingale, widely considered the founder of modern nursing, reduced infection rates among wounded military personnel during the Crimean War when she implemented handwashing and other hygiene practices in her hospital. On the other side of the Atlantic Ocean, Oliver Wendell Holmes, a Boston physician, likewise noticed that infections and mortality could be reduced through handwashing. He correctly hypothesized that hospital-acquired diseases were being transmitted to patients by their physicians via physical contact.

Despite the collective results of these many medical professionals scattered around the world, handwashing was largely dismissed by the scientific and medical communities because no one could satisfactorily explain *why* or *how* an infection could be transferred from one person to another. Even when Louis Pasteur confirmed the existence of microorganisms a decade later—thereby solving the mystery—several more decades would pass before the concept of germs would be accepted by the wider medical community, and antisepsis would be formally adopted as a routine medical procedure.

Why did it take so long for physicians to accept this answer and adopt handwashing? For one, physicians couldn't believe that their existing practices weren't good enough. Medicine had advanced so far so quickly it seemed almost miraculous. The notion that the very same practices that saved lives might, under different circumstances, actually *end* lives seemed inconceivable. On top of that, the idea that the physicians themselves played a role in their patients' infections and deaths, instead of curing them, contradicted the prevailing wisdom of the time and bruised a lot of egos in the process.

Some Treatments Are Better than Others

In many respects, the current state of mental health treatment to prevent suicidal behaviors mirrors the context of the 19th century. Two hundred years ago, the causes of puerperal fever among women giving birth were unknown to the medical community, but evidence from multiple sources suggested that handwashing could reduce fever-related deaths much better than status quo practices. Today, the causes of suicide are similarly unknown, but evidence from multiple sources suggests that certain types of treatments and interventions can reduce suicidal behaviors better than status quo practices, which often conceptualize suicide as a symptom or outcome of mental illness. Consistent with this perspective, status quo practices target a patient's diagnosed mental illness based on the assumption that reducing these symptoms or eliminating the psychological or behavioral disorder also will reduce or eliminate the risk of suicide. If, for example, you are diagnosed with depression, then your clinician might provide therapy to reduce your depression and/or recommend antidepressant medication. As we have discussed previously, though, reducing the symptoms of mental illness does not seem to reduce the probability that someone will make a suicide attempt.

Two treatments in particular—dialectical behavior therapy (DBT) and cognitive behavioral therapy for suicide prevention (CBT-SP)[1]—have demonstrated the ability to reduce the probability of suicidal behaviors in multiple studies conducted by multiple research teams. Other treatments that share many of the same characteristics and components as these treatments—the attempted suicide short intervention program (ASSIP) and mentalization-based psychotherapy (MBP), for example—also have garnered some preliminary scientific support for reducing the probability of suicidal behaviors. Yet another treatment called the Collaborative Assessment and Management of Suicidality (CAMS) also has repeatedly demonstrated the ability to reduce suicidal thinking faster and to a larger degree than status quo treatments. Each of these treatments differs from status quo mental health treatments in one important way: They aim to directly reduce suicidal thoughts and behaviors, regardless of a patient's mental illness, rather than indirectly reducing suicidal thoughts and behaviors by reducing mental illness, the approach taken by status quo treatments. Because DBT, CBT-SP, the crisis response plan (CRP), and CAMS directly focus on suicide risk instead of mental illness, they often are collectively referred to as "suicide-focused treatments."

In 2008, Nicholas Tarrier conducted a meta-analysis of 28 treatment studies to examine how suicide-focused treatments compared to status quo treatments. Tarrier's results showed that individuals who received a suicide-focused treatment subsequently reported significant reductions in suicidal thoughts and behaviors, but suicidal thoughts and behaviors did not change much among individuals who received status quo treatments. Similar results were recently replicated in an even larger meta-analysis conducted by Kathryn Fox and colleagues. In that impressive study, which included over 1,000 treatment studies, Fox found that cognitive behavioral therapies contributed to larger reductions in suicidal thoughts and behaviors than did other types of therapies, including medication only. Fox also found that suicide-focused treatments provided slightly larger benefits than treatments that targeted mental illness. In other words, status quo treatments and suicide-focused treatments were both helpful, but suicide-focused treatments were better.

There is some evidence that these treatments may be getting even better. Since the turn of the century, for instance, patients who receive CBT-SP are at least 50% less likely to attempt suicide as compared to patients who receive status quo treatments. By comparison, in Fox's meta-analysis, the relative risk of suicidal thoughts and behaviors was reduced by only 9% across all published treatment studies, and by 19% across the 52 studies of cognitive behavioral therapies. Patients receiving suicide-focused treatments also report faster reductions in suicidal thinking than patients receiving status quo treatments, but symptoms of mental illness do not necessarily improve at a faster rate. CAMS also seems to do a better job reducing suicidal thoughts than status quo treatments but does not do a better job of reducing suicidal

Table 6.1   Effect of Suicide-Focused Treatments on Symptoms of Mental Illness, Suicidal Thoughts, and Suicidal Behavior

Effect	DBT	CBT-SP	CRP	CAMS
Significantly reduces symptoms of mental illness	✓	✓	✓	✓
Significantly reduces suicidal thinking	✓	✓	✓	✓
Probability of suicidal behaviors is lower than with status quo treatments	✓	✓	✓	
Reductions in suicidal thinking are faster than with status quo treatments		✓	✓	✓
Reductions in symptoms of mental illness are faster than with status quo treatments				✓

behaviors. These general patterns are summarized in Table 6.1, and they suggest that the things that reduce the symptoms of mental illness probably are not the same things that reduce the probability of suicidal behaviors.

Unfortunately, we don't know which "active ingredients" of suicide-focused treatments enable them to reduce the probability of suicidal behaviors better than status quo treatments. We can, however, reasonably conclude that suicide-focused treatments do a better job of reducing the probability of suicidal behaviors because they act upon something other than the symptoms of mental illness. If reductions in mental illness accounted for reductions in suicidal behaviors, we would expect individuals who receive suicide-focused treatments such as DBT and CBT-SP to have larger reductions in these variables than individuals who receive status quo treatments. We also would expect individuals who receive CAMS to have a lower probability of suicidal behaviors than individuals who receive status quo treatment. That's not what we see, though; improvements in mental illness seem to have little (if anything) to do with the reduction of suicidal behaviors in suicide-focused treatments. If mental illness is unrelated to the reduction of suicidal behaviors in suicide-focused treatments, what is the "something else" that these treatments are acting upon? Based on the research reviewed in the previous chapters, I would argue that the "something" involves decision-making processes related to self-regulation. Specifically, DBT and CBT-SP seem to reduce the probability of suicidal behaviors because they strengthen individuals' internal braking systems, helping them to choose *not* to act upon suicidal impulses and urges in stressful situations.

Dialectical behavior therapy

The first suicide-focused treatment to reduce the probability of suicidal behavior successfully was DBT, an outpatient psychological treatment approach developed in the 1970s and 1980s by Marsha Linehan, a clinical psychologist who is arguably one of the most influential suicide researchers of the past century. DBT comprises both individual psychotherapy and skills-based educational groups. Individual therapy sessions and skills training groups are typically scheduled on a weekly basis for six months to a full year, and are organized around four core skill sets involving self-regulatory processes: mindfulness, interpersonal effectiveness, distress tolerance, and emotion regulation (Table 6.2). These core skills are relevant to mental illness, but they are not specific to any particular diagnosis or condition; difficulty observing one's experience without judgment, interacting effectively with others, withstanding or enduring negative emotional states, and identifying and changing one's internal states reflect most (perhaps even all) psychological diagnoses and conditions. These concepts are also key to self-regulation and the capacity to hit the brakes when accelerating toward a collision with suicide. The applicability of these four skill sets across multiple types of mental illness reflects DBT's transdiagnostic, suicide-focused design.

In addition to providing individual therapy—typically scheduled for one hour per week—and group skills training—typically scheduled for one to two hours per week—DBT therapists also provide phone consultation to individuals in-between scheduled therapy sessions. The primary purpose of these phone consultations is to reinforce the use of skills learned in group meetings and individual therapy sessions. Patients consequently spend time

Table 6.2 Four Core Skills of Dialectical Behavior Therapy (DBT)

Skill	What It Is
Mindfulness	The ability to observe what is happening to you in the moment without judgment or self-criticism
Interpersonal Effectiveness	The ability to interact effectively with others, regardless of the type of relationship one has with them
Distress Tolerance	The ability to withstand and endure stress and other negative emotional states
Emotion Regulation	The ability to identify or recognize one's emotions and to change or influence them

during therapy and group sessions learning new skills and how to use them, and then receive help and support to put these skills to use "in real life." A central goal of DBT is for patients to learn how to respond more effectively to intense emotional pain and distress *without* the use of suicidal and self-injurious behaviors. Over the course of treatment, patients learn how to recognize, endure, and change these emotions using alternative strategies. At its core, DBT seeks to alter patients' ability make effective decisions during periods of uncertainty and intense emotional distress and to help them make decisions that improve quality of life.

Since its initial development 40 years ago, DBT has been tested in multiple studies conducted around the world with both adults and adolescents. Over and over again, studies have found that patients who receive DBT are somewhere around 50% less likely to attempt suicide than patients who receive more traditional forms of mental health treatment. DBT also costs much less than other treatments, primarily because it reduces psychiatric inpatient hospitalization and medical treatment costs associated with keeping someone alive or tending to their wounds after a suicide attempt. Because of this long track record of scientific support, DBT is easily the most well-researched and well-studied mental health treatment for suicide prevention. It is, in some respects, the standard against which all other suicide-focused treatments are compared.

The remarkable success of DBT for preventing repeat suicide attempts is tempered to some degree by its complexity. DBT involves multiple components that can require a lot of time from both patients and therapists: weekly individual psychotherapy, weekly group-skills training, and weekly therapist consultation for six months up to an entire year. Furthermore, each of the four DBT skill sets includes dozens of strategies and concepts. On the one hand, this is good because no single strategy is right, and different people are likely to prefer different strategies. On the other hand, all of those different strategies and skills make DBT hard for mental health professionals to learn and challenging for agencies to implement. As a result, many clinicians and agencies provide "DBT-informed" services or "DBT-based" programs, which typically means they are using some, but not all, of DBT's components. The overall effectiveness of these modifications has not been extensively tested, although one recently completed study suggests DBT's skills training groups, during which patients learn concrete strategies for responding to stressful situations, may be more valuable than other parts of DBT. This important finding may explain why Fox's meta-analysis did not find a statistically significant reduction in the risk of suicidal thoughts and behaviors across 29 studies of DBT; DBT-informed or DBT-based interventions may be less effective if they exclude the parts of DBT that are most potent. Just as removing the chlorinated lime from Semmelweis' handwashing solution would reduce its efficacy as an antiseptic, removing components of DBT that teach patients how to recognize one's emotions without judgment, to interact effectively with others, to endure negative emotional states, and to change one's internal states are especially key for reducing the probability that someone will try to kill themselves. A central lesson to be learned from DBT research is that the ability to pump one's internal brakes matters a great deal.

Cognitive behavioral therapy for suicide prevention

The desire to more efficiently reduce the probability of suicidal behaviors influenced the development of CBT-SP in the 1990s and early 2000s by treatment researchers, including David Rudd, Greg Brown, and Aaron Beck. CBT-SP preserves many of the central components of DBT listed in Table 6.2, but delivers them in less time, often in less than six months. Like DBT, CBT-SP focuses on skills training designed to strengthen self-regulation and alter decision-making style, although one slight difference between DBT and CBT-SP is the latter's central focus on teaching skills designed to directly influence and change the patient's belief systems, assumptions, and thought processes that contribute to suicidal behaviors. These include hopelessness (e.g., *Things will never change*), self-hatred (e.g., *I deserve to be punished*), perceived burdensomeness (e.g., *People would be better off without me*), entrapment (e.g., *There's no way out*), and unbearability (e.g., *I can't take this any longer*). Cognitive reappraisal skills training is included within DBT as well, but this particular procedure is a more prominent part of CBT-SP.

Cognitive reappraisal skills are intended to help patients learn how to identify negative and maladaptive thoughts and beliefs that contribute to and sustain suicidal thoughts and behaviors and to help them learn how to replace these thoughts with more balanced and life-affirming beliefs (e.g., *It'll be okay; Just because I make a mistake doesn't mean I'm a failure; This may be difficult but it's not impossible; I can handle it*). These life-affirming beliefs serve to weaken the perceived value of suicidal behavior by strengthening the perceived value of life. In CBT-SP, individuals are taught how to make effective decisions when under duress in uncertain situations; you may not know what's going to happen in the future and you may not always get what you want, for instance, but sometimes we *do* get what we want and things end up going better than expected, so it may be better to make a decision based on that possibility rather than making a decision based on the assumption that things won't work out. In this way, CBT-SP teaches the person to slow down and collect more information before acting.

Early versions of CBT-SP were designed to reduce the probability of suicidal behaviors in approximately six months or less, typically over the course of 20 outpatient individual therapy sessions (one hour per session). Further refinements simplified the treatment even more, leading to even briefer individual therapy formats that now range from 10 to 12 sessions on average. In 2005, a team of researchers led by Greg Brown published the results of a study comparing the effectiveness of cognitive therapy for suicide prevention (CT-SP), one particular model of CBT-SP, as compared to status quo mental health treatment, finding that approximately 24% of patients who received CT-SP attempted suicide during the 18-month follow-up as compared to approximately 42% of the patients who received status quo treatment. CT-SP therefore reduced the probability of suicide attempts by almost half, similar to DBT.

When the results of the CT-SP study were published, many mental health professionals were skeptical that a treatment as brief and simple as CT-SP could be so effective. Another decade would pass before a study of brief cognitive behavioral therapy for suicide prevention (BCBT), a second version of CBT-SP, would be published and provide further support for this treatment model. As luck would have it, I was able to take part in this second study, which was led by David Rudd. In that study, we tested the effectiveness of BCBT as compared to status quo treatment for suicidal military personnel. We started the study in 2010 and enrolled 152 patients over the course of two years, randomly assigning them to receive either 12 sessions of BCBT or status quo treatment and then following them for two years, well after they had finished treatment. At the end of the two-year follow-up period, 14% of the patients who received BCBT had attempted suicide as compared to 40% of the patients who had not—a 60% reduction in suicide attempts that closely mirrored the results of Brown's study conducted nearly a decade earlier.

More recently, a small pilot study was conducted to test the BCBT protocol as adapted by Mark Sinyor and colleagues for use with youths ranging from 16 to 26 years old; the study compared this adapted treatment to status quo group therapy. Twelve youths were randomly assigned to participate in BCBT and 12 were randomly assigned to participate in status quo treatment, and then followed for one year. At the end of the year, none of the youths who received BCBT had made a suicide attempt as compared to three of the youths who received status quo treatment. Although this study was not large enough to make definitive conclusions, the overall pattern nonetheless provides additional support for the value of the BCBT protocol and the CBT-SP approach more generally, and it lent further support to the key lesson learned from DBT: teaching people how to slow down their decision-making while highly distressed can reduce the probability of suicide attempts.

Crisis response planning

While we were still in the midst of our BCBT study, Rudd and I formulated the idea for our next treatment study: testing the crisis response plan (CRP) as a stand-alone intervention for reducing the short-term risk of suicidal behaviors. The CRP is a procedure contained within BCBT that helps suicidal patients to remember how to respond effectively to stressful situations instead of attempting suicide. The CRP contains several key components: (1) recognizing one's personal "warning signs" for an emotional crisis, (2) using simple strategies to reduce one's stress or to distract oneself from the situation, (3) thinking about reasons for living, (4) reaching out to friends, family members, or other sources of social support to reduce one's stress or to distract oneself from the situation, and (5) accessing professional support or crisis services. These components are typically handwritten on an index card so it can be easily carried in a wallet, purse, bag, or backpack.[2] At its core, the CRP is designed to reduce the probability of suicidal behavior with the same process as DBT and CBT-SP: strengthening self-regulation.

Our plan for the CRP study was to compare the effectiveness of this method to status quo crisis management procedures, which typically include a suicide risk assessment interview, supportive counseling, provision of mental health treatment resources, and a verbal contract for safety. This last piece of status quo crisis management, the *contract for safety*—sometimes also referred to as a *no-suicide contract*—is widely-used by mental health professionals. In this procedure, suicidal individuals are asked to agree, whether verbally or in writing, not to kill or injure themselves. The contract for safety focuses on what *not* to do when in uncertain and emotionally overwhelming situations.

The CRP, by contrast, does the reverse: it outlines what *to do* when in uncertain and emotionally overwhelming situations. Going back to our automobile metaphor, the contract for safety encourages suicidal people not to crash their car when speeding toward a brick wall, whereas the CRP teaches them where the brakes are located and how to use them.

In 2012 we received a grant to test the CRP among military personnel who showed up in an emergency room or behavioral health clinic for unscheduled appointments. If a patient reported thoughts about suicide during the past week or a past suicide attempt (whether or not they were currently thinking about suicide), we invited them to participate. Patients who agreed to participate—97 in total—were randomly assigned to receive the CRP or status quo treatment and were then scheduled for ongoing mental health treatment. Our research team followed up with patients for the next six months to assess their suicidal thoughts and behaviors. At the end of the study, only 5% of those who received a CRP attempted suicide as compared to 19% who received the status quo treatment—a 76% reduction in suicide attempts. Within a year of publishing our results, two more studies conducted by two separate research teams found that various iterations of the safety planning intervention, a suicide prevention method that is very similar to the CRP, also reduced suicidal behaviors by 20% to 50% as compared to status quo treatments.

All of these suicide-focused interventions—DBT, CBT-SP, and the CRP—aim to change how a person makes decisions within the context of intense emotional distress and uncertainty about the future. Although these strategies strengthen the individual's capacity to respond effectively to stress and life challenges, they do not go so far as to promise that the individual will experience a life that is completely devoid of stress or problems. On the contrary, a central assumption of these interventions is that adversity is simply a part of living and negative emotions can be natural and useful responses to unexpected, uncontrollable, and unfortunate life events. DBT, CBT-SP, and the CRP focus on teaching individuals how to respond to stressful situations in a more balanced and less extreme manner, thereby helping them to adopt a safer decision-making style and to stick with successful methods even when they occasionally do not work. In many respects, these treatments teach people how to endure the discomfort of waiting for a second marshmallow when you don't know if and when that next marshmallow will become available. They may still experience emotional distress in response to life events, but the magnitude of this stress may be reduced. Many patients who have completed CBT-SP say, for example, that the treatment helps them to "not get so worked up," or to better modulate their emotional distress.

Why Suicide-Focused Treatments Work Better than Status Quo Treatments

Neuroscience research suggests this enhanced ability to self-regulate may be associated with positive changes in brain functioning and connections. Just as germ theory helped physicians and scientists to identify and understand why and how handwashing with chlorinated lime solution reduced infection and mortality rates, the integration of neuroscience research methods into clinical trials could help us to identify and understand why and how suicide-focused treatments reduce suicidal behaviors. There is reason to suspect, though, that the prefrontal cortex and the ventral striatum may be involved. As noted in the previous chapter, these two brain structures appear to be involved in different aspects of decision-making. These are not the only parts of the brain involved in decision-making, though, so it's entirely possible that some other part (or parts) of the brain are affected by BCBT. The brain is a highly complex network of interconnected structures, such that the whole is greater than the sum of its parts. Because of this, and consistent with the notion of emergence, some neuroscientists and other researchers have started to investigate how many different parts of the brain work together instead of just focusing on how a handful of brain structures work in isolation. These interconnected brain structures that work in tandem are referred to as networks. Three neural networks in particular have received a considerable amount of attention: the central executive network, the default mode network, and the salience network.

The *central executive network* involves interconnections among brain structures responsible for information processing, problem solving, and decision-making. The ventromedial prefrontal cortex belongs to this network. The central executive network is active when we are engaged in externally directed thoughts and cognition such as planning ahead, generating options to solve a problem, weighing the pros and cons of these options, selecting a course of action, and inhibiting decisions and actions. The *default mode network* involves interconnections among brain structures responsible for thinking about others, thinking about the self, remembering the past, and planning for the future. The default mode network is active when we are engaged in internally directed thoughts and cognition such as autobiographical memories, thinking about future goals and events, making decisions that involve valued rewards, experiencing positive emotions, and making inferences about others' intentions. Finally, *the salience network* involves interconnections among brain structures responsible for detecting and integrating sensory, emotional, and cognitive information. The ventral striatum, also discussed in the previous chapter, belongs to this network. The salience network tends to be continually active, thereby enabling us to pay attention to what is happening in our environment, how to interpret and understand what is going on around us, and how to coordinate a response to such circumstances.

When these three networks are functioning as intended, the default mode network and central executive network serve complementary roles—a neural yin and yang of sorts—such that when one network is active the other is dormant. The salience network appears to be involved in moderating the switching back and forth between these two complementary networks, especially in response to stressful and uncertain situations. The salience network essentially governs which of the two networks is running at any given time. The default mode network tends to be active when we are at rest and not engaged in purposeful activities, such as watching a television show or a movie, remembering a past event, or allowing our minds to wander. When we need to engage in mentally demanding or goal-directed tasks, however, such as solving a problem or making a decision about something, the salience network activates the central executive network and deactivates the default mode network. Once the mentally demanding task or behavior is complete, the salience network switches things back to the default mode network, shutting off the central executive network.

Among suicidal individuals, several disruptions in the functioning of each network have been identified by researchers. The most consistent findings thus far involve the default mode network and central executive network, both of which appear to have decreased activation levels and decreased interconnectivity among their components. In combination, this hinders each network's ability to do its job effectively. Individuals with disrupted activity in the default mode network and the central executive network are more likely to experience excessive rumination and self-criticism, and struggle to experience and maintain positive emotions, to reduce or control negative emotions, and to inhibit impulses and associated actions. The strategies used in suicide-focused treatments are designed to reverse or counteract these problems.

Newer research has detected changes in brain functioning that line up with these patterns among individuals with post-traumatic stress disorder (PTSD), a condition that is strongly correlated with suicide. Chadi Abdallah, for instance, invited military personnel diagnosed with PTSD to participate in a magnetic resonance imaging (MRI) scan before and after receiving a type of trauma-focused therapy that uses procedures and strategies similar to those used in CBT-SP. Their results showed improved connectivity and activation within the central executive network among those who completed the therapy. Military personnel who received a different type of therapy did not show any improvement in the central executive network, however. Similar findings have been reported by other researchers as well, suggesting that some of the procedures contained in CBT-SP are associated with structural changes within the brain known to be involved in future planning, option generation, and control of emotions and impulses. Although these studies have not yet been conducted with suicidal individuals receiving suicide-focused treatments and interventions, they provide some clues about what might be happening during these treatments.

Within the framework of the cusp catastrophe model of suicide, suicide-focused interventions may be altering the shape of an individual's behavior surface. Specifically, suicide-focused treatments may be increasing the steepness of the slope that connects lower risk states to higher risk states, thereby making it harder to reach higher levels of suicide risk (see Figure 6.1). Before treatment, the behavior surface may have a shallow slope like the behavior surface on the left of Figure 6.1. A ball kicked uphill would roll a greater distance before stopping and reversing directions. Because the slope prior to treatment is so shallow, someone can experience more severe emotional distress and, by extension, higher levels of suicide risk, even in response to an event that isn't particularly stressful. After treatment, however, the behavior surface might have a steeper slope like the behavior surface on the right of Figure 6.1. A ball kicked up this behavior surface would roll a shorter distance before stopping and reversing direction. Here, the very same stressor would result in a much lower level of emotional distress and suicide risk. In addition to reducing the distance traveled by the ball, a steeper hill also causes the ball to return to its starting point much faster. After treatment, individuals with steeper slopes return to lower risk states and lower levels of emotional distress much faster. When conceptualized in this way,

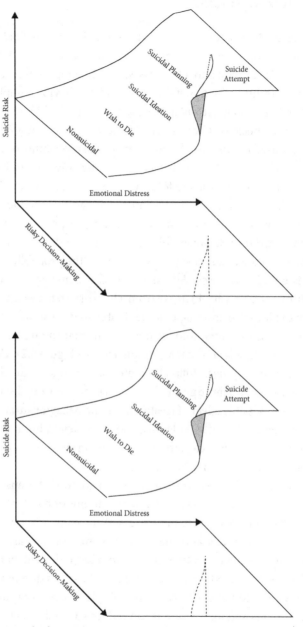

Figure 6.1 Suicide-focused treatments may reduce the probability of suicidal behaviors by altering the slope of the behavior surface. The slope of the behavior surface on the left is relatively shallow and constant across the full length of the surface, whereas the slope of the behavior surface on the right has a much steeper slope towards the right hand side of the surface. A ball kicked from the left edge of each behavior surface to the right has a lower probability of climbing the slope of the surface on the right as compared to the surface on the left. This, in turn, reduces the probability of suicidal behavior.

suicide-focused treatments reduce the probability of suicidal behaviors because they (a) make it harder for a person to reach a high-risk state and (b) make it easier to return to a low-risk state following a stressful situation. This doesn't eliminate the possibility of suicidal behavior completely—if a ball is kicked hard enough it will make it to the top of the hill—but this probability is reduced because it becomes harder to reach that point.

Suicide-focused treatments also may reduce the probability of suicidal behavior by altering the behavior surface in another way, that is, by reducing the size and shape of the double fold. As noted previously, the double fold determines the boundaries of the region of overlap and the location of the tipping point for catastrophic change. If this tipping point is reached, individuals can jump from the lower fold to the upper fold, switching suddenly from a low-risk state to a high-risk state, wherein the probability of suicidal behavior is greatly increased. Suicide-focused treatments may reduce the probability of a catastrophic increase from a low-risk state to a high-risk state by altering the location and shape of the double fold. In some cases, the behavior surface may be altered to such an extent that the region of overlap on the control surface is eliminated completely (see Figure 6.2). Under these circumstances, the tipping point is eliminated and change in suicide risk level becomes smoother and more gradual rather than sudden and discontinuous. Here again, this possible effect of treatment on the behavior surface does not eliminate the possibility of suicidal behavior completely, but it does reduce the probability of a sudden, catastrophic increase in suicide risk among individuals with riskier decision-making styles.

Although suicide-focused treatments seem to work because they impact how a person makes decisions while under emotional duress, we don't yet know for sure if this is actually the case.[3] In many ways, we are in the same boat as Semmelweis and the medical community nearly 200 years ago. Back then, evidence from multiple sources indicated handwashing could reduce fever-related deaths as compared to status quo practices, but no one knew why. Today, evidence from multiple sources indicates suicide-focused treatments and interventions can reduce suicidal behaviors as compared to status quo practices, but we don't really know why. It's possible that decision-making processes will ultimately prove to be the underlying reason, but it's also possible that this hypothesis will prove to be incorrect, just as the concept of miasma was eventually shown to be wrong. If so, that's OK; suicide-focused treatments will continue to work even if we're wrong about

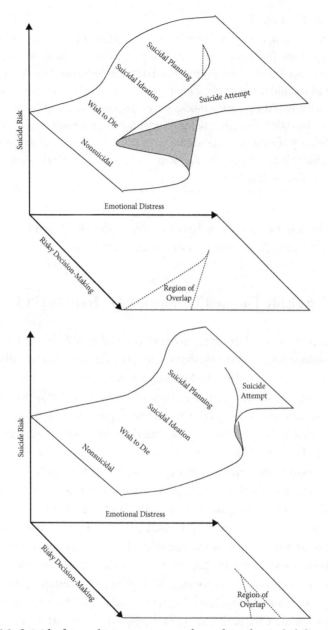

Figure 6.2 Suicide-focused treatments may also reduce the probability of suicidal behaviors by altering the size and location of the behavior surface's double fold. The double fold in the behavior surface on the left is very large, resulting in a large region of overlap that is located in the bottom left region of the control surface. The double fold in the behavior surface on the right is much

Figure 6.2. Continued

smaller, resulting in a very small region of overlap that is located in the bottom right of the control surface. If an individual with a risky decision-making style experienced an increase in emotional distress, they could suddenly jump from the lower fold to the upper fold of the behavior surface when (for the surface on the left) they reach a moderate level of emotional distress or (for the surface on the right) when they reach a very high level of emotional distress. The probability of a catastrophic shift from a low to high risk state is therefore lower for the behavior surface to the right. This, in turn, corresponds to a lower probability of suicidal behavior.

---

the reasons and causes, just as handwashing with chlorinated lime solution worked even though Semmelweis was wrong about why.

Suicide-Focused Treatments Are Hard to Find

This brings us to another similarity between today and the mid-19th century: Despite evidence showing that newer practices can significantly reduce the probability of mortality, the broader medical community has been slow to adopt them. Two hundred years ago, physicians were slow to adopt the practice of handwashing. Today, mental health professionals have been slow to adopt suicide-focused treatments. The slow adoption of suicide-focused treatments is perhaps most evident in the continued use of contracts for safety and no-suicide contracts by mental health professionals despite active discouragement of these methods for at least a decade and a half. In a 2006 paper titled, "The Case Against No-Suicide Contracts," for instance, several prominent suicide researchers provided what is arguably the most comprehensive argument against the use of contracts for safety and no-suicide contracts ever published. In that paper, researchers proposed the CRP as a newer, alternative strategy. Since then, multiple expert consensus panels have similarly recommended against contracts for safety and no-suicide contracts and proposed the CRP and interventions similar to the CRP (e.g., the safety planning intervention) as an alternative.

Despite this, contracts for safety and no-suicide contracts continue to be used by many mental health professionals. Some research has even found that, after receiving training in the CRP or the safety planning intervention, many clinicians continue to endorse contracting for safety as an appropriate suicide prevention strategy, just like physicians continued to insist that their traditional practices were sufficient and appropriate for decades after Semmelweis, Nightingale, and Holmes demonstrated the lifesaving potential of handwashing, and Pasteur proved the existence of germs. Physicians didn't just insist that they were right, they also continued to use status quo practices even after the existence of germs had been proven, their causal role in infections had been explained, and the benefits of using antiseptic agents such as chlorinated lime solution had been shown. Today, more than a decade after researchers first articulated the rationale for abandoning the practice of no-suicide contracts and contracts for safety and multiple studies have shown that suicide-focused treatments worked better than status quo mental health treatments, mental health professionals continue to use status quo procedures anyway. Why?

Inadequate training of mental health professionals

One factor is poor training. A 2012 report from the American Association of Suicidology highlights this issue. Titled, "Preventing Suicide through Improved Training in Suicide Risk Assessment and Care," the report summarizes the findings of a task force convened to review the state of mental health professional training in suicide risk assessment and care practices. Their findings were alarming, to say the least: Fewer than half of psychology training programs, one in four social work training programs, one in 16 marriage and family therapy training programs, and one in 50 counselor education training programs provide *any* amount of education or training focused on suicide as a part of their curriculum. Psychiatry training programs initially seemed to do better—over nine in 10 include some kind of suicide-focused education or curriculum for psychiatry residents—but only one in four of these programs provide *skills-based* training. Skills-based training is critical because this is how clinicians acquire clinical competency; self-guided learning and lecture-based education often is not enough for mental health professionals to become competent in a particular clinical procedure or method. Supervision and oversight by a skilled teacher or instructor is also key.

To illustrate the importance of skills-based instruction, imagine that you require a surgical procedure to address a life-threatening health condition. You consult with two different surgeons to get their opinions and recommendations. The first surgeon tells you they learned how to perform the procedure via hands-on experience under the careful supervision and oversight of another surgeon who had a great deal of experience conducting the procedure. The second surgeon tells you they learned how to perform the procedure by reading textbooks and attending a day-long workshop, but they were never shown how to do it and never received any supervised, hands-on guidance from another surgeon. Which surgeon would you prefer for your life-threatening condition? If you're like me, you would prefer the first surgeon because they received much better training and, as a result, you probably have greater confidence in their competence and skills. Although the second surgeon has received *some* education, they've never been supervised by someone who knows the procedure well and can intervene or correct them if they start to make a mistake or do something wrong. If someone is going to perform a medical procedure on me that could affect my survival and quality of life, I want some assurance that this person knows what they're doing. I wouldn't be surprised if you see things similarly. Although the benefits of skills-based training seems obvious, the majority of mental health training programs in the United States—regardless of discipline or specialty—provide no such training, and very few mental health professionals subsequently receive this type of training at any point during their careers.

The consequences of inadequate training are highlighted by two studies focused on the safety planning intervention, which is very similar to the CRP. In the first study, Jennifer Gamarra and colleagues reviewed the medical charts of 200 suicidal patients to better understand how mental health professionals were completing the safety planning intervention. Gamarra's team found considerable variability in the quality and completeness of the plans. For example, many plans included generic statements that had been copied and pasted, suggesting they had not been customized to the unique needs of the patient. Furthermore, in the majority of cases there was no evidence of ongoing review of the plan, a recommended strategy that serves to reinforce and encourage its use by patients. Because of these trends, the quality of the typical safety planning intervention in that study was low to moderate on average. In the second study, Jon Green and colleagues reviewed the medical charts of 68 suicidal patients and found a similar pattern: Completeness and quality of the safety planning intervention were low on average. Green's study further considered how the completeness and quality of the intervention was correlated with the later occurrence of suicidal behaviors, and found that the probability of suicidal behaviors was reduced only among patients who received higher quality interventions. Incomplete or low-quality safety plans were much less likely to prevent suicidal behaviors. The probability of suicidal behavior was reduced, therefore, when clinicians did a better job using the newer procedure, but the probability of suicidal behavior was higher when clinicians used practices that were closer to the status quo.

In both of these studies, researchers concluded that the safety planning intervention's low quality was likely attributable to inadequate training of mental health professionals. Interestingly, the quality of these interventions remained low despite the creation and easy accessibility of manuals and other training resources online. These resources were not enough, however, to overcome clinicians' limited training and experience. Simply having access to books and materials that described the procedures wasn't enough for mental health professionals to do the newer intervention well. This may seem like an obvious point, but it hasn't yet translated into meaningful change in how mental health professionals are trained. To this day, the majority of mental health professionals receive little to no skills-based training in suicide-focused treatments and interventions. This happens in part because most of the instructors and supervisors affiliated with mental health professional training programs did not receive this training themselves. As a result, status quo knowledge and expertise is passed down to their students, some of whom will eventually become instructors and supervisors themselves and pass down status quo knowledge and expertise again. Even more alarming, however, is how many mental health professionals—up to one in three, according to one study—continue to endorse older, less effective procedures like contracting for safety even *after* they have received training in suicide-focused treatments. Old habits are hard to break.

Dilution of suicide-focused treatments

Yet another problem involves the tendency for many mental health professionals to deviate from the original design and structure of suicide-focused treatments by changing or altering the procedures they were taught to use. Sometimes, these modifications involve the removal of components that were originally included in the treatment. Other times, mental health professionals add components that were never a part of the original treatment. In my experience, mental health professionals often modify suicide-focused treatments so they will "fit better" with what they're already doing, essentially changing them so that they are more similar to status quo practices. Doing this runs the risk of eliminating or diluting the very things that distinguish suicide-focused treatments from status quo treatments and make them so much better. Sure, it's entirely possible that *some* of the modifications that mental health professionals make to suicide-focused treatments can make the treatments even more effective than they are already. When these modifications are not tested systematically, however, we run the risk of rendering a treatment *less* effective, similar to how adding water to antiseptic solutions in order to make handwashing "fit better" with previous practices can actually weaken the formula's life-saving potential.

Even though we know that suicide-focused treatments reduce the probability of suicidal behaviors better than status quo treatments, mental health training programs rarely teach these practices. As a result, mental health professionals rarely use them routinely and suicidal individuals rarely receive them. The treatments that hold the greatest promise for suicide prevention are therefore largely unavailable to those who heed the advice of the suicide prevention community and seek out mental health treatment. To me, this is one of the most frustrating and tragic realities of contemporary suicide prevention efforts: We repeatedly implore people to "get help" because "treatment works," but when someone follows this advice, there is only a remote chance that they will receive one of the better treatments that are currently available. This is not to say that suicide-focused treatments and interventions such as DBT, CBT-SP, and the CRP are right and status quo treatments are wrong. Suicide-focused treatments and interventions are, however, *better* than status quo treatments. Sure, status quo treatments probably reduce patients' symptoms of mental illness and also may reduce their suicidal thoughts, but status quo treatments do not appear to address a key vulnerability that influences the emergence of suicidal *behaviors*: the ability to make balanced decisions while under duress. In that sense, status quo treatments may help someone to take their foot off the accelerator, but when speeding toward catastrophe, people also need to know how to work the brakes.

The Potential Impact of Mental Health Treatment on Suicide Rates

How much impact could a widespread shift from status quo treatments to suicide-focused treatments have on suicide rates? Samantha Bernecker and colleagues recently sought to answer this question in a research study that focused on BCBT, one of the suicide-focused treatments discussed previously. In their study, Bernecker found that for every 100 suicidal patients who received BCBT instead of status quo treatments, one death by suicide could be averted.[4] This may not seem like a particularly big benefit, but if we consider that approximately 1.4 million U.S. adults attempted suicide in 2017, of which half to three-quarters received mental health treatment of some kind, the potential benefits of switching to suicide-focused treatments accumulates very quickly. If all of these adults who received mental health treatment were to receive BCBT instead of status quo mental health treatment, Bernecker's results suggest that somewhere between 7,000 and 10,500 suicide deaths may be prevented, an amount that would reduce the national suicide rate by approximately 15% to 22%. Even in Bernecker's worst-case scenario, which assumed that 500 individuals would need to receive CBT-SP instead of status quo treatment to prevent a single death by suicide, an estimated 1,400 to 2,100 suicide deaths could be prevented, reducing the national suicide rate by approximately 3% to 5%. Given studies of DBT and other forms of CBT-SP have obtained similar results as BCBT, it seems likely that these other suicide-focused treatments would have similar benefits.

Many treatments can reduce the symptoms of mental illness and suicidal thinking, but only a handful of treatments can reduce the probability of suicidal behaviors. These treatments can only have a positive impact, however, if they are embraced by the mental health community and replace the status quo. Two hundred years ago, infection-related deaths could have been reduced and many, many lives could have been saved if the medical community had adopted antiseptic handwashing practices earlier. Full-scale adoption required more than simply knowing and accepting that handwashing could save lives, however; it also required changes to medical school and nursing curriculums to ensure professionals understood why and how handwashing was important, changes to hospital and clinic budgeting and inventory procedures to ensure antiseptic solutions were available on site and remained in stock, and changes to how medical professionals behaved to ensure the actual use of handwashing.

Today, suicidal behaviors could be similarly reduced via the adoption of suicide-focused treatments by mental health professionals, but it also will take a multipronged approach that targets the knowledge and behavior of individual mental health professionals, the content of mental health training programs, and the ways in which healthcare systems operate. Change of this type would require the involvement of each mental health discipline's accrediting bodies and licensing boards. Mandating educational curriculum and skills-based training in suicide-focused treatments is one way to achieve this goal, although this will almost certainly be met with resistance. An alternative approach would be to use reward or incentive programs that teach suicide-focused treatments, perhaps by providing them with special designations or benefits such as reduced fees for accreditation renewal or longer accreditation windows. State licensing boards also could require mental health professionals to complete coursework or training focused on suicide-focused treatments. Simply encouraging or mandating the *completion* of suicide-focused curriculum is unlikely to be enough, however; strategies that incentivize the adoption and actual *use* of these treatments and practices without modification also would be helpful. For example, discounts on professional insurance policies and/or licensure renewal fees could be provided to mental health professionals who are able to demonstrate competency in suicide-focused treatments, similar to how home insurance policies and automobile insurance policies offer discounts when our homes and cars have certain safety features known to reduce the probability of adverse events such as fires or accidents. Yet another way to potentially incentivize the use of suicide-focused treatments is for health insurers and third-party payers to provide higher pay and reimbursement rates for mental health professionals who use these specialized treatments and procedures as intended instead of using status quo treatments.

Distinguishing the effects of administrative and clinical practices

Along these lines, we should also take a hard look at the systems and institutions within which clinicians practice. Over the past few decades, healthcare systems and clinicians have increasingly adopted suicide-focused practices and policies intended to improve suicide-risk screening and management practices. On the one hand, this encouraging development reflects a broader commitment to suicide prevention within the healthcare system. On the other hand, these efforts do not always achieve their primary intent of improving the quality of care for suicidal patients. On the contrary, in many instances these efforts create the illusion of improving quality while actually serving to further solidify status quo practices. In my experience, this happens because healthcare institutions typically approach this issue from a legal perspective wherein suicide-focused policies are adopted and certain practices are encouraged because they will presumably reduce the institution's legal vulnerability in the event of an undesired outcome, namely a patient's death by suicide. The usual result of these process-improvement efforts is a uniquely legal one: more forms and more paperwork.

Process-improvement efforts, therefore, tend to focus on changing *administrative* practices rather than *clinical* practices. The typical rationale for taking this approach is that a primary problem facing the institution entails inadequate documentation of suicide risk-management practices by its clinicians. Through the implementation of new forms and additional documentation practices, institutions (and individual clinicians) can ensure that standard of care expectations have been met, which reduces the probability of being sued in the event of a patient's death by suicide. Central to this argument is the notion of "standard of care." Clinicians often assume that the standard of care is a medical and/or scientific concept, but it's not; it's a legal concept that refers to the practices and procedures that a minimally competent clinician in the same field would use under similar circumstances. Said another way, the standard of care can be understood as status quo practice. This is a key point to understand: the standard of care is defined as what a typical clinician *would* do in a given situation, not what a typical clinician *should* do in that situation. Unfortunately, this distinction is often confused, resulting in a potential disconnect between the administrative practices implemented by an institution and the clinical practices actually used by clinicians.

This gap between administrative and clinical practice is reflected in the aforementioned research by Gamarra and Green, who found that the completeness and quality of suicide-focused interventions by mental health professionals were quite low despite institutional implementation of standardized forms, documentation templates, and policies intended to encourage (and enforce) the use of a recommended suicide-focused clinical practices. Administrative changes like these certainly provide the appearance of improved clinical practice and often prompt (or compel) clinicians to change how they fill out forms and document their interactions with patients, but these administrative actions do not necessarily change the thing that actually leads to reductions in suicidal behaviors: good clinical practice and decision-making. Under these circumstances, clinicians continue to use status quo methods while also filling out more paperwork and changing the language used to describe these status quo methods. Because the paperwork and altered language aligns with standard of care expectations, clinicians and administrators are lulled into the false belief that true change in clinical practice has occurred when in reality no change has occurred. Status quo practices have not been replaced by suicide-focused treatments and best practices like those discussed in this chapter; instead, they have been concealed beneath paperwork.

Imagine if a similar approach had been adopted by hospitals and physicians in response to Semmelweis's research. If it had, we probably would have seen hospitals taking steps to craft and develop policies mandating the use of handwashing with antiseptic solutions prior to delivering babies. Hospitals also might have mandated the use of new forms for physicians to fill out for each of their patients who showed up to the obstetrics unit in labor. The forms might have included lists of risk and protective factors for dying of puerperal fever, and probably would even have included a section for the physician to describe how they washed their hands with chlorinated lime solution. Some hospitals may even have distributed information about chlorinated lime solution and the hazards associated with delivering a baby soon after having had contact with cadavers in the autopsy room. The hospital may have stored information and resources about these topics in a central area that could be easily accessed by physicians and all other hospital staff. Hospitals would not have actually purchased any chlorinated lime solution for their staff members, however, and would not have placed any solution next to sinks and handwashing stations. Hospitals also would not have taken any steps to ensure that physicians were actually washing their hands with antiseptic solutions. They would have just checked the medical records to see if physicians were filling out the mandated forms saying that they had done so. It's certainly possible that *some* physicians would have started washing their hands with chlorinated solution, but it's also likely that *most* physicians would have just kept on doing what they had always been doing, albeit under the veneer of good documentation.

Under these conditions, expectant mothers would have continued to contract puerperal fever and die at high rates, however, despite the implementation of good policies and good documentation practices because forms and paperwork do not actually prevent infection-related mortality—antiseptic practices do. Sure, good policy and good documentation might inspire some clinicians to adopt better clinical practices, but this is unlikely to happen if they are not given the tools and resources needed to abandon old practices in favor of newer and better methods. If a hospital does not purchase chlorinated lime solution, does not make it available to its staff, and does not take the time to ensure that staff use these tools appropriately, however, patients will not benefit from these newer practices. On the contrary, patients could actually be *harmed* because administrative change without practice change could create the faulty impression that antiseptic handwashing procedures do not work after all.

This is, in many respects, the current state of affairs of our mental healthcare system. Typically engendered by fears surrounding litigation, efforts to improve care for suicidal patients have emphasized change in administrative procedures without an accompanying change in clinical practice. Changing policies and paperwork is easy; changing the behaviors and actions of clinicians, by comparison, is really, really hard to do. At the end of the day, what matters the most is whether physicians actually wash their hands with antiseptic solutions and mental health professionals actually use suicide-focused treatments. If we want to tackle the wicked problem of suicide, we must make it easier for mental health professionals to learn suicide-focused treatments and make it easier for them to use these treatments as a matter of routine practice, thereby increasing the likelihood that individuals seeking mental health treatment will benefit from them.

In the end, if the suicide prevention community and society more broadly are going to continue encouraging people to seek out mental health treatment when feeling suicidal, we need to make sure that they have easy access to suicide-focused treatments. Status quo practices simply are not enough and need to be replaced by newer methods that yield better results. It's not good enough to stick with what we've been doing for decades, or to stick to what we learned when we were in graduate or medical school; newer solutions that work much better are available now. Replacing status quo mental health treatments with suicide-focused treatments and interventions such as DBT, CBT-SP, and the CRP would likely lead to significant and meaningful reductions in suicide rates.

Even this change, however, would represent just one element of comprehensive suicide prevention, and it is not enough in and of itself. If we want to have a larger and more meaningful impact on suicide, we also need to identify and implement strategies that extend beyond the mental healthcare system.

7

Seat Belts and Second Chances

The modern automobile was first invented in the late 1800s, but it wasn't until the development of mass production methods in the early 1900s that cars started to become widely available to Americans (Figure 7.1). As the number of drivers and cars rapidly increased in the following years, the rate of traffic fatalities also increased (Figure 7.2). This isn't particularly surprising; without cars or drivers, there would be no traffic fatalities. For many years, traffic fatalities also were positively correlated with the distance (or amount) that cars were driven. Here again, this correlation isn't very surprising: spending more time on the road introduces more opportunities for an accident to occur. If you spend only a few minutes per day driving because you live very close to work, your risk for a traffic fatality is much lower than someone who spends a lot more time driving because they have a very long commute. Spending less time in your own car and spending less time around other cars reduces the probability that you will get into a collision, whether caused by you or by someone else.

In the early 1960s, the U.S. traffic fatality rate increased for almost a decade concurrent with several social trends involving motor vehicles: cars became bigger and faster, the interstate highway system expanded, and speed limits increased. These changes increased traffic fatalities because the combination of bigger cars and faster speeds increased the forces involved in collisions; being hit by a very large truck traveling at 60 miles per hour is much more dangerous and potentially lethal than being hit by a compact car traveling at 25 miles per hour. Traffic fatalities started to decline again during the early 1970s due in part to a nationwide reduction in the maximum speed limit, which served to reduce the force of collisions. This change in speed limits was not motivated by the desire to reduce traffic fatalities, however; it was motivated by politics. Specifically, reduced oil production overseas motivated politicians to decrease energy consumption. Once the energy crisis ended, people resumed driving more and traffic fatalities started rising again.

Since 1980, the traffic fatality rate has steadily decreased, falling by almost half despite a steady increase in the number of drivers, number of cars, and

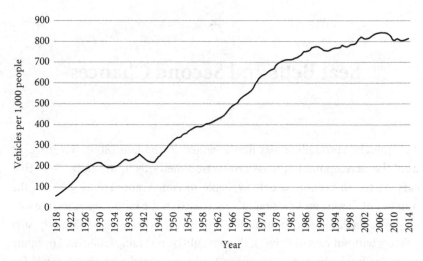

Figure 7.1 Estimated number of vehicles driven on U.S. roads, by year. (Source: Davis, 2019).

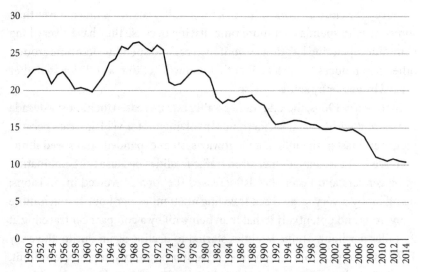

Figure 7.2 Rate of traffic fatalities in the U.S., by year. (Source: National Safety Council, 2019).

number of miles driven by Americans—the opposite of what we would otherwise expect. People were driving more than ever but there were fewer fatalities. In contrast to the decline in traffic fatalities observed during the energy crisis of the 1970s, this more recent drop in fatalities was the result of multiple efforts intentionally designed to achieve this goal, such as building safer cars, designing safer roadways, criminalizing drunk driving, and mandating seatbelt use. Critically, this overall decline in traffic fatalities occurred despite our inability to predict who will die in a traffic accident and when someone will get into an accident. Even with all of the advanced technology and computational methods available to us today, nearly 100 years after cars were first mass produced we are still unable to reliably predict when any traffic accident will occur, fatal or not. There are simply too many variables at play. Sure, we've identified plenty of risk factors for traffic fatalities: male gender, younger age, alcohol use, and faster driving speed (to name just a few), but no combination of these, or other, variables can provide us much information about who will get into an accident or when an accident will occur. We also recognize that each of these risk factors may be causally related to some traffic fatalities to some degree, but none of these variables are causally related to *all* traffic fatalities. Speeding while under the influence of alcohol may contribute directly to some accidents, but sometimes people who speed while under the influence of alcohol do not get into an accident and sometimes people who drive slowly while stone cold sober get into accidents.

Traffic fatalities result from complex interactions among many, many different variables, including driver characteristics (e.g., young age, driving fast), vehicle characteristics (e.g., size of the vehicle, vehicle design, safety features), and environmental circumstances and context (e.g., poor weather conditions, limited visibility). Each of these variables can contribute to traffic accidents and influence the probability that a traffic accident will be fatal. In addition, each of these variables can compound or—conversely—mitigate the effects of other risk factors. Traffic fatalities can be caused by many different things, and there's really no way of knowing when each of those things will (or will not) lead to a tragic outcome for any particular person at any particular time. In this sense, understanding the causes of traffic fatalities is just as complex as understanding the causes of suicide, and determining who will die in a traffic accident is just as impossible as determining who will die by suicide. Despite all this complexity and uncertainty, though, we've done a really good job as a society of reducing traffic fatalities.

A Two-Step Approach to Fatality Prevention

We've achieved this by embracing complexity and resisting the temptation to focus on only a small number of correlates of traffic fatalities. Traffic fatalities cannot be predicted in advance with any reliability, and we don't really waste much time trying to develop algorithms or alert systems to accomplish this goal. On the contrary, we simply accept this reality and focus instead on two related goals: (1) reducing the probability of *all* traffic accidents and (2) reducing the probability that unpreventable traffic accidents will result in death. The logic of the first goal is pretty straightforward: because some traffic accidents are fatal, reducing the occurrence of all traffic accidents in general will also reduce or eliminate those traffic accidents that result in death. The logic of the second goal takes a somewhat different approach, though: reducing the probability that a traffic accident results in death "converts" or "switches" a fatal traffic accident to a nonfatal traffic accident. In essence, the second goal serves as a backup to the first goal. We obviously would like to avoid or prevent *all* traffic accidents from occurring, but some accidents will still occur despite our best efforts, so we also need ways to protect people when our efforts have failed.

With respect to the first goal—preventing someone from getting into any traffic accident—we use a range of educational strategies designed to improve driving skills (e.g., driver's education classes), but this has been nowhere near as successful as measures that have little to no impact on driver traits or ability. For instance, legislative bodies have passed laws that penalize decisions and behaviors that increase the probability of a traffic accident: drunk driving has been rendered a criminal offense and fines are imposed on drivers who engage in unsafe driving practices such as speeding and using cell phones. We also have employed economic and financial incentives to reduce the probability of traffic accidents: auto insurance companies, for example, provide discounts for purchasing vehicles with built-in safety features such as blind spot warning systems. In some cities and jurisdictions, reductions in traffic accidents have also been achieved by altering the design and construction of roadways: The diverging diamond interchange design, which eliminates left-hand turns that cut across traffic moving in the opposite direction, reduces accidents by more than half as compared to the traditional four-way intersection design. At intersections of minor roadways, roundabouts and traffic circles also have been used to reduce the frequency of accidents. None of these strategies influence a driver's skill or ability. Nonetheless, they significantly reduce the likelihood of traffic accidents.

With respect to the second goal—reducing the lethality and severity of traffic accidents—our most successful measures also have virtually nothing to do with driver skill or ability. Government bodies have passed laws that require the manufacture of cars that meet minimum safety standards as well as laws that penalize drivers for failing to use certain safety devices such as seatbelts. Car manufacturers also have designed, tested, and improved a range of safety features, such as air bags and crumple zones, and have increasingly included them as "standard features" in newer car designs. None of these strategies prevent traffic accidents from occurring, but they reduce the likelihood that a vehicle occupant will die should an accident occur. Wearing a seatbelt, for instance, reduces the probability that someone will die in a traffic accident by almost half despite having absolutely no impact on any of the many, many risk factors that contribute to traffic accidents: inclement weather, poor road conditions, limited visibility, human error, speeding, and so on. Air bags, crumple zones, and seatbelts are not designed to impact these factors, though; their sole purpose is to increase the probability of surviving a traffic accident that could not be successfully prevented.

The seatbelt, in particular, has had an enormous impact on traffic fatality rates, but its life-saving potential can only be realized if people choose to buckle up while driving. As we discussed in the previous chapter, getting people to change their behavior—even when the change is really minor and simple—can be very difficult. Nonetheless, our efforts to motivate seatbelt use have been very effective. In the early 1980s, only one in six people wore a seatbelt regularly. To increase seatbelt use, public health experts designed and implemented an aggressive education campaign aimed at changing social norms about seatbelt use. Two decades later, in the early 2000s, almost five in six people were wearing a seatbelt regularly. As seatbelt-use rates started to climb, traffic fatalities started to drop. Today, the percentage of people who wear a seatbelt regularly is even higher—over nine in 10—and the traffic fatality rate is even lower.

Seatbelt use was an important part of reducing traffic fatalities, but it was not the sole contributor to this change; at around the same time, a significant cultural shift involving the (un)acceptability of driving while under the influence of alcohol also occurred. The shift in social norms surrounding drunk driving was prompted in part by the Harvard Alcohol Project, a public health communication and education campaign that was aimed at reducing alcohol-related traffic fatalities. The centerpiece of this education campaign was the "designated driver," a concept that had been developed in Europe but was, at the time, largely unknown to Americans. As a testament to the campaign's success, nearly 30 years later, the concept of a designated driver is now widely recognized within the United States. The Harvard Alcohol Project was not the only effort at that time focused on reducing alcohol-related traffic fatalities; the Ad Council's "Friends Don't Let Friends Drive Drunk" campaign, which similarly targeted social norms surrounding driving while under the influence of alcohol, was launched at around the same time. Of note, these complementary efforts were not intended to reduce or eliminate alcohol consumption; they were instead intended to reduce the number of intoxicated and impaired drivers on the road. This is an important distinction. Recognizing that convincing people to reduce or eliminate alcohol consumption probably would not result in much behavior change—people would probably continue to drink alcohol with little change—the designated driver campaign encouraged safe decision-making instead. If you're going to drink, plan ahead so that your drinking does not cause a traffic fatality. Likewise, if you *don't* have a designated driver but drink anyway, know that other options are still available to you so that you don't drive, such as calling for a taxi or calling a friend.

If the campaign had focused on reducing alcohol consumption itself, it would have likely been ignored by the general public. It also would have missed the central problem of alcohol-related traffic fatalities. Alcohol consumption by itself does not contribute to either traffic accidents or fatalities; choosing to drive while under the influence does. Context matters. At its core, the campaign conceptualized alcohol consumption as a context within which certain decisions could potentially be fatal. This subtle but important shift in perspective almost certainly contributed to the considerable success of the designated driver campaign. Since the early 1980s, the rate of alcohol-related traffic fatalities has shrunk by more than half. Because alcohol-related traffic fatalities account for a large percentage of all traffic fatalities, this reduction in one particular type of fatality has had a pronounced effect on the overall decline observed during the past few decades.

In contrast to the considerable effects of improved vehicle and road design, seatbelt use, and reductions in drinking and driving, improvements in surgical and medical procedures have had a much smaller impact. This is not to say that advances in medicine have had no impact on survival rates among those involved in severe traffic accidents; if you receive medical care after a severe traffic accident today, you are much less likely to die than you might have been several decades ago. Despite this, the size and scope of the benefits from improved medical care pale in comparison to the size and scope of the benefits from these other strategies. This is because improved survival due to medical care requires you to not only survive the accident in the first place, but also to remain alive long enough to get to a hospital where those medical advances can be used. Medical and surgical advances have certainly helped to reduce traffic fatality rates, but this particular measure has had a much smaller impact, relatively speaking, than the aforementioned measures that reduce the probability and lethality of traffic accidents. Said another way, if you are in a severe accident, wearing a seatbelt will influence your overall chance of survival to a much greater degree than the medical care you eventually receive at the hospital. As the saying goes, an ounce of prevention is worth a pound of cure.

Preventing Suicide Without Knowing
Who Will Attempt Suicide

The many strategies described above align with the concept of prevention (or safety) through design. Prevention through design assumes that injuries, illnesses, and fatalities can be most effectively reduced or controlled by designing and building systems that eliminate or remove potential hazards from the very beginning, before they can cause any harm. Prevention through design also assumes that injuries, illnesses, and fatalities are most effectively reduced by targeting the source of the hazard itself. In other words, if a thing is harming people or poses a threat to people, then the best method for protecting people is to get rid of that thing. If complete elimination of the hazard is not possible, though, the next best method is to substitute or replace the hazard with something else that is less dangerous or harmful. If substitution is not possible either, then the next best strategy is to limit people's exposure to the hazard by restricting access or otherwise isolating people from it. If that is not possible, the next best strategy is to impose rules or policies designed to control people's behavior in ways that minimize the likelihood of being harmed. Finally, if none of the previous strategies are possible, the final (albeit least effective) strategy is to issue equipment designed to protect people from the hazard.

This sequential approach to injury and illness prevention is known as the hierarchy of controls and is often displayed as an inverted triangle (see Figure 7.3). Although prevention through design and the hierarchy of controls are most often applied to occupational settings to minimize work-related injuries, the fundamental principles underlying these concepts can be applied in many different areas and domains of life. As applied to traffic fatalities, for instance, crash avoidance systems (e.g., headlights and taillights, rearview mirrors, and braking systems) serve as elimination strategies because they remove potential hazards; designated drivers and safer roadway designs (e.g., traffic circles, diverging diamond interchanges) serve as substitution strategies because they replace more dangerous situations with less dangerous situations; concrete barriers and guardrails serve as engineering strategies because they restrict our access to potential hazards; traffic laws and the many rules of the road that we follow (e.g., speed limits, traffic lights and traffic signs, criminalization of drunk driving) serve as administrative controls because they change or control driving behaviors; and seatbelts and air bags serve as personal protective equipment because they reduce the severity of

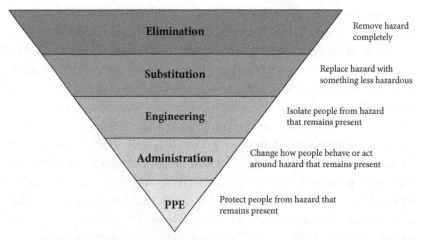

Figure 7.3 The risk for suicide among U.S. adolescents who live in households with a firearm is significantly increased as compared to adolescents who live in households without a firearm. This heightened risk is disproportionately carried by adolescents without a mental illness. Whereas adolescents with a mental illness living in a household with a firearm are 3 times more likely to die by suicide, adolescents without a mental illness living in a household with a firearm are 12 times more likely to die by suicide.

injury and reduce the likelihood of fatality when a hazard is present (e.g., traffic collisions).

Note how the most effective strategies for reducing traffic fatalities, corresponding to the higher levels of control (i.e., elimination, substitution, isolation), largely entail strategies that are primarily intended for changing the *environment* within which traffic fatalities occur rather than changing individual drivers: ensuring that vehicles are designed and built with certain safety features and designing and building roadways to minimize collisions. Even at the lower control levels, which are geared toward changing driver behaviors, the strategies used to enact these changes nonetheless largely focus on the environment: traffic laws are instituted and enforced at the community level (each driver is not, for example, assigned to a police officer who watches their every move) and personal protective equipment is built into our vehicles rather than distributed to individual drivers.

The environmental focus of traffic fatality prevention efforts—and prevention through design approaches more generally—is based in large part on the fact that it is incredibly difficult to know who will be injured, fall sick, or die as a result of hazard exposure, or when a bad outcome such as this might occur. As compared to all of the people exposed to a given hazard, very few get injured, sick, or die. Lots and lots of people drive, for example, but relatively few get injured or die in a traffic collision. Because we can't know with any amount of certainty when a hazard will result in injury or death, it's better to take precautions all the time. Wearing a seatbelt every time we drive ensures that we are protected even when an unpredictable and unforeseen event occurs—someone crashing into us, for instance. Environmental approaches to injury and mortality prevention also help to overcome the tendency for humans to be unreliable and inconsistent in their actions and decision-making. Drivers do not always wear seatbelts, do not always use a designated driver, and do not always obey posted speed limits and follow traffic laws. For these reasons, it is much better to remove hazards, make hazards less dangerous, and/or keep people away from hazards. If we take these steps, we can still reduce the risk of injury, illness, and death even when individuals make unsafe decisions or behave in unsafe ways, and even when we have absolutely no idea when, where, or to whom a traffic accident will occur.

Suicide prevention has historically taken a very different approach. Instead of seeking to change environmental and contextual hazards that contribute to suicide, our efforts have by and large focused on methods designed to change the individual. If a person is suicidal, we recommend mental health treatment. If a person is *not* suicidal but is experiencing stress and/or other risk factors for suicide, we recommend mental health treatment as well. Even when we talk about "public health" approaches to suicide prevention, mental health treatment continues to play a prominent and central role. Universal suicide risk screening, for example, is touted as a critical public health solution for suicide prevention, because expanded screening would help us refer people to mental health treatment. We also encourage people to be alert for suicide warning signs, almost all of which involve mental health concepts, and then encourage people with these warning signs to access mental health treatment or other forms of crisis services (for example, calling a suicide prevention hotline or going to a hospital). All roads lead to mental health treatment and services that are focused on changing the individual. Very rarely do we talk about changing the environment in ways that could eliminate or mitigate factors that contribute to suicide. If we were to apply this same approach to traffic fatality prevention, what might that look like?

Our public education campaigns would probably emphasize the warning signs of fatal traffic accidents. This warning signs might include things like speeding, drifting out of a lane, swerving, fishtailing, intoxication, talking on the phone, and skidding. Our public education campaigns also would probably direct us to encourage these drivers to attend driver education programs and safe driving classes so they can learn driving strategies to minimize these problems and protect them from traffic collisions. We might also advocate for widespread and routine screening of driving ability whenever someone renews their vehicle registration or driver's license. This screening might include questions that ask drivers if they have recently driven faster than the posted speed limit, drifted out of their lane, swerved, fishtailed, driven while drunk, talked on the phone while driving, or skidded out of control while driving. Drivers who positively endorse these experiences would be encouraged to attend driver's education and safe driving classes. If a driver endorsed a lot of these experiences or talked about especially extreme instances of each, we might have them meet with a driving specialist to determine if the driver needed to be forcibly enrolled in these classes so we could improve their driving ability.

We would not expect such an approach to have a meaningful impact on traffic fatalities. This approach would be even less effective if we instituted it without requiring car manufacturers to design and build cars with headlights, taillights, rearview mirrors, turn signals, seatbelts, or brakes; without installing traffic lights, guardrails, or lane dividers; and without enacting any laws or rules to dictate which side of the road we should drive on or how fast we should drive. All things being equal, driver's education and safety classes would probably benefit, at least to some degree, those who voluntarily participated. In the grand scheme of things, efforts to change individual drivers' abilities would have a relatively smaller impact than all of the environmental changes that could have a much larger impact. If this approach seems ridiculous, that's because it is. Nonetheless, this is exactly how we approach suicide prevention.

Injury prevention and suicide prevention efforts also differ substantially with respect to stakeholder engagement. Consider, for example, how injury prevention advocates have worked with policymakers to enact legislation and pass laws designed to influence the behavior of the many groups and individuals who influence traffic fatalities in some way: individual drivers (e.g., setting speed limits, prohibiting drunk driving, mandating seatbelt use), car manufacturers (e.g., setting safety standards), and even the service and hospitality industries (e.g., requiring bartenders to limit or refuse the sale of alcohol to severely intoxicated individuals). These laws and standards affect *all* drivers, not just high-risk drivers. In contrast, when suicide prevention advocates work with policymakers, legislators, and other stakeholders, efforts have largely focused on strategies that center on mental healthcare services and programs—funding mental health treatment services, implementing suicide-risk screening tools, and supporting "gatekeeper" trainings designed to teach about suicide warning signs and to encourage help-seeking behaviors. Yes, researchers have been reasonably successful in developing treatments that can reduce the probability of suicidal behaviors and potentially even reduce the number of suicide deaths, but mental health treatment alone is not enough, just as driver's education and safety classes are not enough to prevent traffic fatalities.

Traffic fatality prevention efforts have invested relatively few resources for developing tools and methods intended to identify who will get into a traffic accident or die in one, but an enormous amount of time and energy has been invested to develop tools and methods intended to determine who will attempt suicide and who will die as a result. These divergent pathways are not attributable, however, to differences in what we know about the correlates of traffic fatalities and the correlates of suicide. Numerous risk factors for traffic fatalities have been identified by researchers, just as numerous risk factors for suicide have been identified. Likewise, the known risk factors for traffic fatalities are no stronger or weaker than the known risk factors for suicide.

This divergence in approach seems to be related instead to our assumptions about the importance of risk identification and detection methods. On the traffic fatality side, we don't expect that any algorithm will ever be able to tell us when and where any driver will experience a traffic accident, let alone die in a traffic accident, and we generally do not anticipate or expect that any algorithms or tools will ever be developed for this purpose. When it comes to suicide, however, we assume that detection and identification methods are critical or even *necessary* for prevention, and we generally expect that suicide-risk screening methods and algorithms should be able to do so.

If we shifted our mindset surrounding suicide prevention in a way that better aligned with the prevention-through-design approach underlying traffic fatality prevention, we might reconsider the considerable time, effort, and resources being devoted to the development and implementation of suicide-risk identification and detection methods. We might consider instead the potential impact of redirecting these efforts toward environmentally focused strategies that are more likely to reduce suicide rates. Just as we've been able to significantly reduce traffic fatalities without knowing which drivers are fatigued, intoxicated, or inclined to reckless driving, we can almost certainly reduce suicides without knowing who has been thinking about suicide or who has various risk factors for suicide.

This is not to say that risk detection methods are completely worthless and have no place in prevention efforts; knowing which drivers are intoxicated can obviously be helpful for determining whose keys should be taken away, thereby reducing the probability of a traffic fatality. Most of us, however, don't know which drivers are intoxicated at any given time, and our limited knowledge about this particular risk factor does not thwart the effectiveness or value of driving a car with headlights, having concrete barriers and guardrails on our roads, installing traffic lights and stop signs at intersections, and wearing a seatbelt. Our lack of knowledge about who is driving under the influence also does not reduce the utility of crumple zones, air bags, and other automobile safety features. Detection and identification strategies can certainly be helpful, but they aren't as essential for preventing traffic fatalities as these environmental and design-based approaches. In like fashion, suicide-focused detection and identification strategies probably aren't as essential for preventing suicide as we have long assumed. Unlike injury-prevention approaches, however, we have not invested much time or resources in implementing solutions that seek to eliminate, substitute, or isolate environmental hazards that contribute to suicide.

Preventing Suicide Without Preventing
Suicide Attempts

Traffic fatality and suicide prevention also differ with respect to how they understand and conceptualize various types of outcomes of interest. Traffic fatalities typically result from traffic accidents, but the majority of traffic accidents do not result in a fatality—for every person who dies in a traffic accident, for instance, 176 survive. Likewise, suicides result from suicide attempts, but the majority of suicide attempts do not result in death—for every person who dies as a result of a suicide attempt, more than 30 survive. To reduce traffic fatalities, we have sought to achieve two goals: (1) reducing traffic accidents and (2) reducing the lethality of traffic accidents that could not be prevented. Traffic accidents can be reduced with higher level controls such as diverging diamond intersections, traffic circles, and collision detection systems. Despite these and other measures, however, some accidents will still occur. Therefore, we complement these strategies with personal protective equipment designed to increase the survivability of traffic accidents: airbags and seatbelts, for instance. Unfortunately, suicide prevention efforts have historically focused on only the first goal: reducing suicide deaths by reducing all suicidal behaviors. No strategy or technique can possibly prevent *all* suicidal behaviors, however. Because of this, we should expend more time and effort on the second goal as well—the suicide prevention equivalent of airbags and seatbelts. Luckily, a reasonably straightforward and simple method for achieving the second goal—reducing suicides by decreasing the lethality of suicide attempts—already exists: means restriction.

Means restriction includes environmental strategies and measures designed to eliminate, substitute, or limit access to potentially lethal methods for suicide, such as certain medications, bridges, toxic substances, and firearms. Means restriction works not by changing anything about people; rather, it works by changing the environment to increase safety, consistent with the prevention-through-design philosophy. Means restriction accomplishes this via the two processes. First, means restriction can block a person's ability to make a suicide attempt by completely removing the method from the environment (i.e., an elimination control) or by blocking or restricting a person's access to the method (i.e., an engineering control). Means restriction is therefore akin to a designated driver. Just as removing an intoxicated person's access to their car reduces the probability of the intoxicated person crashing their car while driving, means restriction removes the suicidal person's access to methods that could be used for a suicide attempt. An intoxicated person can't crash their car if they don't have a car to crash, and a suicidal person can't attempt suicide if they don't have a method for the suicide attempt.

Of course, there's still a possibility that a suicidal person who doesn't have access to one particular method (e.g., a firearm) will just pick a different suicide method instead (e.g., medications). Research suggests this doesn't happen very often—most people actually do *not* switch methods when one method has been restricted. Nonetheless, it's a possibility and probably happens in some cases. Under these circumstances, means restriction functions as a substitution control by replacing a more dangerous hazard with a less dangerous hazard, akin to traffic circles, which restrict drivers from making turns that cross through opposing lanes of traffic and run the risk of head-on collisions. Collisions can still occur in traffic circles, but these collisions tend to be much less severe than head-on collisions because all vehicles are moving in a single direction. Dangerous head-on collisions are thereby replaced by less dangerous collisions.

From a prevention-through-design perspective, the effectiveness of means restriction for preventing suicide hinges on a method's overall lethality profile and its frequency of use. If a particular method has a low lethality profile—meaning it is unlikely to result in death—then limiting access to that method won't make much of a difference, even if the method is used very frequently. Conversely, if a particular method is rarely used in suicide attempts, then limiting access to that method won't make much of a difference either, even if the method is very dangerous and highly lethal. Means restriction therefore works only for methods that are both highly lethal and frequently used. In the United States, only one method currently meets both criteria: firearms. Firearms are both highly lethal—over 90% of those who shoot themselves die as a result—and are frequently used—more than half of all U.S. suicides result from self-inflicted gunshot wounds. In other nations, firearms do *not* meet these criteria, but other suicide attempt methods do. Means restriction therefore needs to accommodate the unique hazards associated with each environment. Again, context matters.

Preventing suicide by making it harder to die by suicide

In Britain, for example, a leading suicide method prior to the 1960s was suffocation via domestic gas, which contained a high percentage of carbon monoxide. Individuals would turn on the gas supply to their home (for example, by turning on the stove), and then breathe the gas until they died. Beginning in the 1960s, however, the carbon monoxide content of domestic gas was steadily decreased in response to new legislation, until it was virtually free of carbon monoxide nearly a decade later. Because carbon monoxide was removed from domestic gas, this change amounted to an elimination control. As the toxicity of domestic gas declined, so did the nation's suicide rate. From 1963 to 1970, the percent of domestic gas that was carbon monoxide dropped from approximately 12% to 0% and the suicide rate dropped from around 14 per 100,000 to 10 per 100,000—a nearly 30% reduction. This decline in Britain's overall suicide rate was almost entirely explained by reductions in carbon monoxide poisoning; suicide by all other methods did not change at all for men and increased by a negligible amount for women. By and large, people who would have died of carbon monoxide poisoning therefore did not die by suicide using a different method. As noted before, it's certainly possible that some individuals attempted suicide using a different method. There's no evidence to suggest this is true, but for the sake of argument let's assume it is. In this case, restricting carbon levels did not prevent *all* suicide attempts from happening, but if any suicide attempts did occur, the elimination of carbon monoxide rendered them much less dangerous and increased the likelihood of survival.

Similar patterns have been seen in rural areas of Asia and the Pacific Islands, where pesticide self-poisoning was a leading cause of suicide for many decades. In Sri Lanka, for instance, suicides increased by nearly eightfold from 1950 to 1995, with nearly two out of three suicides resulting from pesticide ingestion. This problem was closely tied to farming and agricultural communities, where pesticides were used as a tool in day-to-day work and were therefore readily available. When upset or distressed, someone simply had to walk to the storage room, open a bottle of pesticide, and drink it. In response to rising suicide rates, the government of Sri Lanka started to ban the most toxic pesticides in the 1980s and 1990s. These restrictions coincided with a nearly 50% drop in suicides, due almost entirely to decreased instances of pesticide self-poisoning. As the number of suicides from pesticide ingestion dropped, suicides resulting from all other methods remained unchanged, however, suggesting the vast majority of people did not replace pesticides with a different suicide method. Researchers also found that the observed reductions in Sri Lanka's suicide rate did not coincide with change in any other risk factors commonly associated with suicide, such as unemployment, alcohol consumption, and divorce rates. The only variable that consistently correlated with the decline in suicides was banning highly toxic pesticides. The government did not ban *all* pesticides; just the ones with especially toxic chemicals and additives. Their approach to means restriction aligned with a substitution rather than elimination control.

Sri Lanka is not alone in achieving this remarkable feat; in Samoa, suicides increased nearly fivefold from 1975 to 1980 after pesticides containing the highly toxic paraquat chemical were introduced to the nation, but the suicide rate reversed direction and dropped by almost two thirds after new legislation controlling the sale of paraquat was implemented in 1980. Here again, substituting a more toxic pesticide with less toxic pesticides reduced suicide deaths. This change may not have prevented *all* suicide attempts. It seems entirely possible that some farmers drank the newer, less lethal pesticides—but they weren't dying as a result of doing so.

What about medications? Means restriction works here, too. In the United Kingdom, suicide rates dropped after legislation was passed in 1998 to reduce the maximum package size for paracetamol, an over-the-counter pain medication—an engineering control approach that restricted or limited people's exposure to lethal amounts of the medication. In Australia, restrictions on the availability of barbiturate medications in the late 1960s were followed by a marked reduction in overdose suicides and overall suicide rates. In Denmark, multiple elimination controls were employed to address several different methods of suicide, leading to reductions in suicide rates: barbiturate prescriptions declined in frequency, legislation mandating the removal of carbon monoxide from car exhaust was passed, improved safety features designed to prevent the release of carbon monoxide in households were introduced, and restrictions on an opioid pain killer called dextropropoxyphene were imposed. In all cases, there were no increases in the use of other methods of suicide, suggesting means substitution did not occur.

What about jumping from heights? Means restriction works. The installation of bridge barriers and safety fences—an engineering control strategy—has been associated with dramatic reductions in jumping suicides from bridges located around the world: the Clifton suspension bridge in Bristol, England; the Ellington Bridge in Washington, DC; and the Memorial Bridge in Augusta, Maine, to name just a few. The *removal* of such barriers is also associated with the reverse pattern: *increased* suicides. When a safety barrier designed to prevent jumping suicides was removed from the Grafton Bridge in Auckland, New Zealand, for instance, the number of suicides from that bridge increased fivefold. After a new barrier was reinstalled five years later, the number of suicides dropped back to zero. Another interesting finding about jumping-related suicides is that when a barrier is erected on a bridge, jumping suicides typically do not increase at other bridges located close by. Therefore, people do not go to a different bridge because their first choice was thwarted; they simply don't jump. Here again, switching methods (or in this case, locations) has not been supported.

What about firearms? Means restriction works for that, too. Arguably the best example of this here in the United States occurred in the District of Columbia after the Firearms Control Regulation Act was enacted in 1976. The law required residents of the District of Columbia to maintain a registration certificate in order to possess a firearm and to register their firearms within 60 days of the law's implementation, both of which represent administrative controls; any firearms that were not registered during this time frame were deemed illegal and could not be registered thereafter. The law also required that registered owners store their firearms either locked up or unloaded and disassembled, two types of engineering controls. Soon after the law took effect, firearm suicides dropped by 23% but the number of suicides by all other methods did not change—people were not switching to a different method. Researchers further showed that suicides in neighboring Maryland and Virginia counties—jurisdictions that were not subject to the law's provisions—did not change during the same period of time, thereby ruling out the possibility of other naturally occurring shifts in suicide rates within the region. The law's effect on suicide, therefore, was limited to those who were subject to it.

A similar pattern was observed in Israel after its military instituted a new policy requiring soldiers to leave their government-issued firearms on base when going home for leave on the weekends, an elimination control method. Prior to 2006, there were approximately 28 suicides per year on average in the Israeli military, of which 26 (93% of all suicides) were due to firearms. In many cases, these suicides occurred during the weekend and involved government-issued firearms, which were taken home by soldiers during weekend leave. After the policy change was enacted, however, suicides among Israeli military personnel dropped by 40%, mostly because the number of firearm suicides dropped without much change in suicides involving other methods—no evidence of switching means.

Other lines of research further support the life-saving effects of laws and policies designed to reduce access to firearms. In U.S. states with more laws that are designed to strengthen background checks (administrative control), improve child safety (engineering control), ban military-style assault weapons (elimination control), and restrict firearms in public places (elimination control), suicide rates are much lower than in states without these laws. The effect of these laws on suicide rates is surprisingly strong. In states with mandated waiting periods for the purchase of firearms (administrative control), background checks (administrative control), open-carry restrictions (elimination control), and gun lock requirements (engineering control), suicide rates are approximately 25% to 40% lower than in states without these laws. This reduction is due in large part to differences in firearm suicide rates. In states with these laws, firearm suicides are approximately 45% to 70% lower than in states without these laws. Of these various types of laws, requiring handguns to be locked up in at least some circumstances seems to have the strongest correlation with reduced suicide rates. Interestingly, firearm legislation may have a stronger influence on suicides than it has on homicides, a trend that reflects the little-known fact that two thirds of all firearm-related fatalities in the United States are suicides. This is an especially noteworthy statistic when considering the extent to which public discourse surrounding firearm deaths and firearm legislation focuses on homicide with little to no attention directed toward suicide.

Taken together, the many, many studies supporting the effectiveness of means restriction provide very strong evidence that suicides can be prevented through environment-oriented, prevention-through-design approaches. These methods prevent suicide without suicide-risk screening, without suicide-risk detection systems and algorithms, and without mental health treatment, all of which are best categorized as personal protective equipment controls because they seek to mitigate risk and harm when in the presence of an environmental hazard. Mental health treatments can change how people respond to their environment, but they can't change the environment that surrounds them. Mental health treatments are therefore akin to seatbelts and airbags: they're good to have and definitely reduce the probability of severe injury and death when you get into an accident, but a much better solution would be to avoid the accident in the first place. Along these lines, the potential benefits of means restriction routinely dwarf the potential benefits achieved from treatment-oriented solutions. In the previous chapter, we discussed how widespread adoption of suicide-focused treatments could, in the best-case scenario, potentially reduce the national suicide rate by up to 15% to 22%. Means restriction, by comparison, reduces suicide rates by margins that consistently range from 30% to 60%—nearly double the estimated impact of improved mental healthcare.

Preventing suicide by reducing firearm availability

Here in the United States, where firearm suicide is especially common, the notion of means restriction often comes with considerable discomfort and anxiety owing to the politically contentious nature of gun control. It's important to note, however, that means restriction does not necessarily have to take the form of banning or completely restricting firearms; reducing easy and immediate access to a loaded firearm via engineering controls would likely have a positive effect. Supporting this possibility is research showing that the presence of a firearm in a home increases the probability that someone living in that home will die by suicide, but this risk can be mitigated when these firearms are stored in certain ways. For example, David Grossman and colleagues found that although the risk of suicide is several times higher for children who live in households with a firearm than for children who live in households without a firearm, this difference is reduced greatly if the firearm is stored unloaded and locked up, the ammunition is locked up, and/or the firearm and ammunition are kept in separate locations—all of which constitute engineering controls. Using *any* of these strategies—even only one—was associated with a greater than 50% reduction in firearm suicides among children. Suicides were also lower when both the firearm and its ammunition were inaccessible to the children; the use of lockboxes and gun safes to store firearms, for instance, was associated with very large reductions in suicides among children.

The protective effects of safe storage practices are not limited to children, though; these same patterns also have been seen among adults. A study by Edmond Shenassa found that people who died by firearm suicide were more likely to have a firearm in their home, but safe storage practices, an engineering control, reduced this risk. Shenassa's results also suggested that the protective effect of locking up a firearm and keeping it unloaded was very strong for gun owners who had *fewer* risk factors for suicide. For those with multiple risk factors, however, safe storage did not seem to confer as much protection, suggesting the life-saving benefits of safe storage practices are

strongest for individuals *without* obvious signs or indicators of mental illness. Two separate studies conducted by David Brent and Arthur Kellermann
arrived at similar conclusions. In Brent's study, the presence of a loaded
firearm in a home increased the risk of suicide among adolescents *without*
a mental illness by 12 times but did not increase the risk of suicide among
adolescents *with* a mental illness (see Figure 7.4). In Kellermann's study, the
discrepancy was even more dramatic: The risk of suicide was 33 times higher
among individuals (including both adults and children) *without* a history of
mental illness but was only three times higher among individuals *with* a history of mental illness.

Over and over again, across methods and nations, limiting the availability
of suicide methods that are both highly lethal and commonly used has been
associated with reductions in suicide rates. Indeed, at a population level,
means restriction is the *only suicide prevention strategy that consistently reduces suicide rates*. Despite this singular distinction, means restriction has
not played a central role in U.S. suicide prevention efforts, and has routinely been placed on the back burner even though firearms and suicide in
the United States cannot be meaningfully separated from each other. When
firearm safety and means restriction more generally *are* discussed, suicide
prevention advocates have tended to couch their benefits within the context
of acutely suicidal or "high risk" individuals with a mental illness. Although
focusing on high-risk individuals is intuitive because these individuals have
the highest probability for engaging in suicidal behaviors, this approach is
essentially the *opposite* of what scientific studies suggest would be most effective and useful.

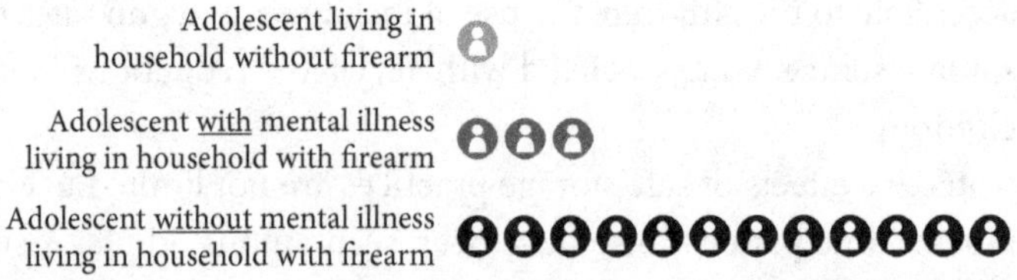

Adolescent living in   😐
household without firearm

Adolescent <u>with</u> mental illness   😐😐😐
living in household with firearm

Adolescent <u>without</u> mental illness   😐😐😐😐😐😐😐😐😐😐😐😐
living in household with firearm

Figure 7.4 The risk for suicide among U.S. adolescents who live in households
with a firearm is significantly increased as compared to adolescents who live in
households without a firearm. This heightened risk is disproportionately carried
by adolescents without a firearm. Whereas adolescents with a mental
illness living in a household with a firearm are three times more likely to die by
suicide, adolescents without a mental illness living in a household with a firearm
are 12 times more likely to die by suicide.

In Shenassa's study, people who died by firearm suicide reported fewer symptoms of depression than did people who died from other causes even though they were also more likely to have recently experienced a negative change in employment (e.g., demotion, job loss, quitting a job). This pattern mirrors CDC data: suicide decedents without a mental illness are more likely to have experienced a recent life stressor and to have used a firearm than suicide decedents with a mental illness. These various lines of evidence suggest that firearm-oriented means restriction methods such as safe storage practices will probably have the greatest protective effect on people *without* mental illness who are experiencing an acute stressor as compared to people with mental illness. Comprehensive suicide prevention, therefore, should encourage safe firearm storage practices among *all* gun owners, not just those who have a mental illness and/or other risk factors for suicide. After all, we require *all* vehicles to be built with certain safety features and encourage *all* drivers to wear a seatbelt every time they drive, not just those who are "high risk" and not just when someone is driving in high-risk conditions. Just as wearing a seatbelt can reduce the risk of dying in an unexpected collision, using a locking device can reduce the risk of dying during an unexpected period of intense emotional distress.

Safe firearm storage practices could reduce suicide via one of two possible mechanisms. First, safe storage practices could slow someone down enough during periods of intense emotional arousal when a risky decision-making style can be especially dangerous. The extra time required to unlock and/or load the firearm under these circumstances may provide just enough time, even if only seconds or minutes, for someone's emotional arousal to drop just enough that he or she shifts back to a lower risk state and can identify and select an alternative action. Safe firearm storage does not prevent someone from getting into a high-risk state, but it does render the high-risk state less dangerous and buys the individual some extra time to take their foot off the accelerator and hit the brakes. Even if their forward momentum can't be stopped completely, it may be slowed enough to reduce the severity of any suicidal behavior that does occur.

Second, safe storage may decrease an individual's "cognitive access" to firearms. Cognitive access refers to the psychological appeal or prominence of a potential method for suicide. Individuals who are thinking about suicide and have ready access to firearms, for instance, are more likely to assume that they will someday act upon these thoughts and urges. In a recent study, Lauren Khazem and colleagues examined this possibility by considering how firearm storage and various aspects of suicidal thinking were correlated with each other. In that study, Khazem asked the participants, all of whom were firearm owners, how they stored their firearms at home. Their responses revealed that those who used safe storage practices were just as likely to think about suicide as those who did not use safe storage practices. Among participants with recent suicidal thoughts, however, those who did not use any safe storage practices were more likely than participants who did use safe storage practices to say that they expected to attempt suicide someday. Individuals with easily accessible and loaded firearms at home were more likely to view suicidal behavior as a possible outcome in their future.

These findings remind me of a suicidal patient who received psychological treatment from a graduate student I once supervised. The patient had firearms at home, so the student asked him to describe his firearm storage methods and safety procedures. Over the course of the conversation, the patient agreed that placing all of his loaded weapons in a gun safe was a good idea, at least while he was engaged in treatment. Once treatment was finished, they agreed to revisit the issue to discuss whether it would be safe to remove these safety precautions. After a few weeks without his firearms readily available, the patient reported that he was no longer thinking about suicide and commented that locking up his firearms, where they were out of sight, made a big difference. "Every time I would see one of my guns," he said, "I would think about killing myself and felt like I had to fight against those thoughts." Once he placed all of the firearms in his safe, however, he found himself thinking about suicide much less often. Although the firearms were still located in his home, they were—in his words—"out of sight, out of mind." Relatively small changes in firearm storage practices, therefore, could serve the same purpose as taking your foot off the accelerator. It may not slow you down as much as the brakes, but at least you're not accelerating anymore.

I suspect the same is true for other possible methods for suicide as well, especially for people who experience on-again, off-again suicidal thoughts and urges. Seeing things in the environment that could be used for suicidal behavior—knives, medications, and ropes, for example—may activate suicidal thoughts for some people. Removing or limiting access to these things via one or more environmental control strategies could reduce the probability of injury or death. This possibility aligns with research showing that individuals who pay more attention to things associated with death and suicide are more likely to make a suicide attempt, as well as the personal accounts of individuals who have experienced persistent thoughts of suicide.

This general pattern probably extends beyond potential suicide methods. Eliminating or limiting our access to things in our environment that elicit suicidal thoughts and urges can be especially useful or powerful strategies for suicide prevention. Unfortunately, environmentally oriented, prevention-through-design methods receive comparatively less attention from the suicide prevention community than strategies and methods designed to change people.

The Importance of Second Chances

A significant reason for our lack of progress in suicide prevention relates to our hyperfocus on mental illness, which has narrowed our thinking about suicide so much that we overlook the fact that suicides also occur among individuals *without* mental illness. We focus so much of our effort on trying to figure out *who* is going to kill themselves and trying to thwart the reasons *why* someone would want to kill themselves that we haven't spent much time thinking about *how* people kill themselves. Means restriction methods work irrespective of the potential causes of suicide, and do not depend on our ability to predict who will attempt suicide or when suicidal behaviors will occur. Instead, means restriction focuses directly on reducing the lethality of suicidal behaviors, thereby increasing the likelihood that someone will survive a suicidal crisis, giving them a second chance.

The importance of having a second chance cannot be understated. Of those who survive a suicide attempt, the vast majority report feeling relieved that they were alive and regret making the attempt. Across 90 research studies that have followed suicide-attempt survivors for up to 10 years, around seven out of 10 people who attempted suicide and survived did not attempt suicide again and nine out of 10 did not go on to die by suicide. If someone survives their first suicide attempt, there's a very good chance that they will not die by suicide at all, even many years later. Firearms and other highly lethal methods rob the individual of this second chance. We cannot prevent all suicidal behaviors from ever occurring, no matter how hard we try and what methods we employ, because we cannot prevent people from ever experiencing intense periods of acute emotional distress and cannot always influence the decisions they make in those circumstances. Stress is a natural and normal part of the human experience that can occasionally become so extreme that it is uncomfortable, even painful, to endure. Scientists have identified a range of strategies that individuals can use to better endure these emotional states and/or to reduce the negative impact of these emotions on our lives, but even these strategies won't work all the time. Ensuring that people survive their first suicide attempt is an incredibly important objective for suicide prevention. We need a backup plan that offers a second chance.

In the 1980s, traffic fatalities started to drop despite the increased number of drivers and cars on the road because we focused on changing the environment that surrounds drivers instead of changing the drivers themselves. Suicide prevention needs to follow suit. To accomplish this, we must shift our focus toward eliminating or reducing environmental hazards that contribute to suicide. One promising method for accomplishing this is means restriction. In the United States, such an approach implicates an increased emphasis on firearms. This approach will require us to engage government officials and gun manufacturers about the need for safer firearm designs and safer storage methods, just as we have done to build safer cars and safer roads. We also need to change social norms surrounding firearm storage practices and allowing trusted individuals to temporarily hold onto firearms during vulnerable periods, just as we have done to increase the use of seatbelts and designated drivers.

To achieve these aims, the suicide prevention community will need to overhaul its communication and outreach strategy. Messaging that adopts an injury prevention approach and emphasizes the cultural values and principles of gun owners has the potential to be much more successful than traditional approaches that emphasize concepts and themes surrounding mental illness. Such messaging could, for example, highlight the importance of protecting Second Amendment rights while also protecting oneself and one's loved ones from unnecessary harm. It also could emphasize the importance of safe storage practices such as temporarily reducing access to firearms during difficult times. Furthermore, instead of presenting safe storage practices as a suicide prevention measure, safe storage practices could be presented as a characteristic of proud, responsible, and safe gun owners. Recent research by Elizabeth Marino and colleagues found that gun owners were more willing to temporarily remove firearms from their homes, to temporarily hold a friend's firearms, to speak with a friend or healthcare professional about temporarily holding their own firearms, and to give their firearms temporarily to a trusted individual after hearing messages framed in this way as compared to gun owners who received traditional suicide prevention messages focused on warning signs and treatment-seeking behavior. Culturally sensitive messages informed by a prevention-through-design mindset can make a big difference.

I'm not convinced that the complete elimination of firearms is a realistic or achievable goal in the United States, at least not at any point in the near future, but increasing the rate of safe storage practices among gun owners by changing social norms surrounding firearm safety *can* be achieved. In less than two decades we dramatically reduced traffic fatalities without spending much time or effort trying to improve driving ability. I'm confident we could achieve comparably dramatic reductions in suicide deaths if we were to reframe our efforts to reduce suicide and use an injury-prevention perspective instead of the mental illness viewpoint that has dominated our thinking about suicide for decades. Prevention-through-design strategies will not (or cannot) eliminate *every* suicide—wicked problems can't be solved with any single strategy—but they can expand the range of interventions that are likely to have a positive impact.

8

Creating Lives Worth Living

Reducing firearm availability would go a long way toward reducing the U.S. suicide rate, but it would have little to no impact on those who do not own or have access to firearms, and it would not necessarily prevent suicide by other methods. Targeting multiple environmental hazards that increase the risk of suicidal behaviors is necessary to maximize the likelihood of impacting the many different types of individuals who are vulnerable to suicidal behavior. For example, research by Alex Gertner and colleagues suggests that reducing economic insecurity by increasing the minimum wage could reduce suicide. In their study, which tracked suicide rates and state minimum wage levels from 2006 to 2016, U.S. states with higher minimum wages had lower suicide rates overall. On top of this, whenever a state's minimum wage increased, the state's suicide rate slowed in the following year by approximately 1% to 2% for each $1 per hour increase. For many Americans, raising the minimum wage could either remove or reduce the hazards of economic insecurity and financial strain, and thereby may reduce their risk for suicide, even if only slightly.

In a different study, Leonardo Tondo and colleagues found that suicide rates were higher in U.S. states with higher proportions of uninsured citizens, fewer physicians, and lower spending on mental healthcare. Conversely, Matthew Lang showed that when a state passed laws requiring mental health benefits to be included and equal to physical health benefits in health insurance plans, the state's suicide rate dropped by approximately 5%. Among those with a current or recent mental health diagnosis, health insurance coverage does not increase the likelihood of receiving mental health treatment, however, suggesting that merely *having access* to health insurance and mental health treatment coverage, whether or not these benefits are actually used, may be the most important factor, possibly because access to these benefits reduces the psychological hazards associated with worry about the rising cost of health care. Making health insurance more accessible could reduce suicide rates by a few more percentage points.

Environmental physical-health hazards warrant attention, too. Amanda Bakian and colleagues identified a positive short-term correlation between air pollution levels and suicide during a 10-year period of time, with elevated levels of nitrogen dioxide and fine particulate matter in the air being significantly associated with increased rates of suicide two to three days later. Similar results have been seen around the world in a variety of nations with a wide diversity of weather patterns, geography, and cultures, providing some confidence that the pattern is not simply a fluke. The reasons for this relationship are not yet known, but Bakian's team has hypothesized that high levels of nitrogen dioxide and fine particulate matter may reduce oxygen levels and increase inflammation of the brain. Reducing the number of days with high levels of nitrogen dioxide, particulate matter, and sulfur dioxide in the air—something that can probably only be accomplished through legislative action—could potentially reduce suicide rates by a few percentage points.

Although the potential benefits of the strategies implicated by these studies are admittedly quite small—suicides may only decrease by one to two percentage points for each additional $1 increase in the minimum wage, for each additional 1% of the population who has health insurance, and for each additional day without high air pollution—in combination they could add up. More importantly, though, these strategies address social and environmental hazards that cannot be remedied with mental health treatment. Mental health treatments can help people gain a different perspective on these problems and make different decisions when under duress, but they can't increase people's income or eliminate their credit card debt or provide them with health insurance or pay the mortgage or make their boss less of a jerk or make their parents accept their sexual identity. We can encourage people to access mental health treatment to prevent their suicide, but what is a person to do if their suicidal crisis is driven by debt and financial strain, underemployment and housing insecurity, discrimination and oppression, workplace harassment and bullying, or domestic abuse? These sources of emotional stress are not mental illnesses, and mental health professionals have little to offer beyond providing support and resources. If we want to prevent suicide effectively, we need to look beyond the individual. Context matters.

Preventing Suicide by Improving Quality of Life

Of the many patients who have helped me to recognize the importance of context, Jenny impacted me the most. I first met Jenny when she was in her mid-twenties. She was referred to our clinic by Todd,[1] an acquaintance whom my wife and I had met through our suicide prevention work. Jenny had been struggling with post-traumatic stress disorder (PTSD) ever since she had been sexually assaulted several years earlier. Todd was aware of a new two-week treatment program we had developed for military personnel and veterans struggling with PTSD. In this program, which we called the R&R Program, military personnel and veterans diagnosed with PTSD or sub-threshold PTSD (which means having all but one of the required symptoms of PTSD) received individual cognitive processing therapy (CPT) on a daily basis from a mental health professional who had received extensive training in the method. In the decades since its initial development, CPT has garnered very strong scientific backing as a treatment for PTSD. Because of this considerable body of scientific support, CPT is one of only a handful of treatments recommended by the Department of Defense, Department of Veterans Affairs, the Institute of Medicine, and other expert panels for the treatment of PTSD.[2]

One of the central ideas of CPT is that PTSD can be understood as stalled recovery. Stalled recovery refers to the fact that when any of us experiences or witnesses a dangerous or potentially life-threatening event, such as a physical assault, sexual assault, combat, or a motor vehicle accident, it is natural to feel jumpy and on edge, to think about the event a lot, to experience negative emotions such as anger and anxiety, and to avoid situations that remind us of the event. These reactions are natural because they are designed to protect us; if we are harmed or almost harmed in a situation, these "symptoms" of PTSD are essentially our brain's way of telling us to be careful so we can minimize the risk of being harmed again in the future when in similar situations. As time passes, these natural reactions will gradually decline in intensity and frequency for most of us; we think about the event less often, we resume activities we had temporarily given up, our anxiety lessens, and our sleep improves. These changes occur because of built-in self-regulatory mechanisms designed for the purposes of recovery.

Most of us will go through this natural recovery process after a stressful event, but a smaller number will follow a different path over time. Some, for instance, will continue to experience uncomfortable emotions such as anxiety, guilt, and anger, and continue to have unwanted and uncontrollable thoughts and memories about the event. Others, however, will not experience a pronounced reaction right after the event but will start to experience it at a later time, sometimes many years later. PTSD occurs when these otherwise natural reactions and experiences worsen and spread to other areas of life, such that we are no longer avoiding just the situation in which we experienced harm or potential harm; we also start avoiding other people, places, or circumstances that remind us of that original situation. Avoidance can even generalize to other situations that bear little resemblance to the original event; we don't feel comfortable in crowded areas such as shopping malls, concerts, or movie theaters, for instance, even though the original event occurred in a completely different location—a combat zone, on the highway, or at home. When this happens, recovery stalls and we become "stuck." We can get stuck for many different reasons, but CPT generally focuses on the role of unhelpful thoughts and beliefs, based on the assumption that what we tell ourselves about the event and how that event has impacted us can contribute to getting stuck and staying stuck. In CPT, we seek to identify these unhelpful thoughts and beliefs, consider the ways in which they are unhelpful, and then identify ways to develop and adopt other, more helpful perspectives. As these newer perspectives are learned, people get unstuck, kick starting the recovery process that had been stalled for so long.

The onset of Jenny's PTSD occurred during her first year of college after she was sexually assaulted by a male acquaintance. Jenny reported the incident almost immediately to her roommate, friends, parents, university administrators, and law enforcement. Instead of providing support, however, just about everyone in Jenny's life responded with disbelief or criticism. Why was she studying with this guy alone? Why did she accept his invitation to walk her back to her dorm? Was she sexually active with other men? When did she first lose her virginity? Why didn't she fight back harder to defend herself? Did she understand how an allegation like this could negatively impact the accused and the university? Was she *sure* that the sex wasn't consensual? In the face of this onslaught, Jenny started to blame herself for the rape and to criticize herself. I should've known, she told herself. It was my fault. I should've fought back. I've ruined my life. I can't control my emotions. I'm crazy. I can't make good decisions. I'm worthless. No one cares about me. Things will never work out for me. Soon thereafter, Jenny started experiencing the tell-tale symptoms of PTSD: unwanted memories and dreams about the assault, refusing to talk about it with anyone, avoiding situations where she might be alone with men, and intense shame, self-blame, anger, and anxiety. Jenny considered leaving the university but felt trapped. She had a scholarship that completely covered the cost of her tuition; if she transferred to another school, however, she probably would not receive any scholarship at all. Stuck between a rock and a hard place, Jenny chose to stay put. She stopped talking about the event with everyone in her life, even her own family, who "didn't really know what to say or how to react." Jenny learned it was better to just avoid the topic all together.

Not long after graduating, Jenny moved away from home, hoping to put her past behind her. It wasn't that easy, though. She continued to experience intense guilt, shame, and self-blame, and struggled to form and maintain meaningful and supportive relationships with others, especially men. Jenny's life during these years was marked by frequent change: moving multiple times, switching jobs, and entering and exiting multiple relationships. Jenny sought out and enrolled in a variety of treatment programs that included different types of individual and group therapy, meeting with multiple therapists and counselors over the years. According to Jenny, these various treatment experiences helped "a little bit," but "we never really got at the heart of the issue." Over time, Jenny become increasingly hopeless about the future, which seemed bleak and full of unending despair. She no longer experienced positive emotions like happiness and hope, and she found it difficult to enjoy activities and events that used to be pleasurable and exciting. Jenny started thinking about death and suicide. If this is all that life is going to be, she wondered, then what's the point of living?

Todd was familiar with Jenny's struggles and had watched her slowly decline over time. Todd asked if we would be willing to help Jenny, and we agreed to do so. After years of struggling with PTSD and years of receiving therapy with little to no benefit, Jenny was understandably skeptical that any more treatment could possibly help, let alone a program as brief as two weeks, but Todd convinced her to give it a shot. Jenny eventually decided to attend the program, and arrived a few weeks later. "I figured I'd try one more time," she later told me, after we had finished treatment. If the treatment didn't work, she reasoned, she could always kill herself instead.

During treatment, Jenny identified her unhelpful thoughts about the rape, learned how to evaluate these thoughts, and identified and tried out a number of alternative perspectives. Perhaps there was no way to know in advance that the rape was going to happen. Perhaps the rape wasn't her fault after all. Perhaps her decision not to fight back, motivated by a self-protective desire to minimize the violence and aggression directed toward her, was a reasonable one to make in that circumstance. Perhaps her decision to stay at the university was well-reasoned instead of self-destructive. Perhaps her anger with her parents, her friends, the university administration, and the criminal justice system was justified. Perhaps she really could experience happiness and joy in life again. After a few days of daily CPT, when we were not yet halfway through the treatment, Jenny tearfully reported that she was feeling something she assumed had been lost forever: hope.

The techniques used in CPT—which are designed to teach people how to recognize and identify unhelpful thoughts, to examine them from different perspectives, to generate alternative perspectives, and to select the option that works best within a given situation—are also used in brief cognitive behavioral therapy (BCBT), one of the versions of cognitive behavioral therapy for suicide prevention (CBT-SP) that we discussed in a previous chapter. Both CPT and BCBT use the same techniques to help people gain perspective, although the focus of these techniques differs slightly; in BCBT, the primary focus is thoughts and beliefs related to suicide, whereas in CPT, the primary focus is thoughts and beliefs related to trauma. Of course, suicide-related beliefs and trauma-related beliefs overlap a lot and have a great deal in common—self-blame and self-criticism, for instance, are shared by individuals with PTSD and individuals who are contemplating suicide. Many of us who use these two treatments in our clinical practice often find ourselves addressing both suicide-related and trauma-related beliefs, no matter which treatment protocol we happen to be using. This overlap probably explains why patients who receive CPT experience significant reductions in suicidal ideation—a pattern we've seen now in multiple studies.[3]

During the course of treatment, patients start to see themselves, others, and the world in a new light. Perhaps you're not a burden on others. Perhaps making a mistake is different from being a complete and total failure. Perhaps the situation is not as unbearable as you think. Perhaps things won't end up as bad as you expect. Perhaps you don't have to act upon your suicidal thoughts after all. Perhaps you actually do deserve happiness, joy, and respect. As these new perspectives emerge during the course of treatment, so, too, does hope. "Maybe that light I see ahead of me in the darkness isn't a train bearing down on me after all," one patient said to me when he was halfway through CBT-SP. "Maybe it's the light at the end of the tunnel."

These changes in perspective appear to coincide with changes in brain structure. As you may recall from Chapter 6, the central executive network is responsible for integrating information about what's going on around us, the emotions we experience, our expectations about future consequences, and how we decide to act. Multiple response options can be generated and evaluated within the context of these various information sources. Once a response option is selected, alternative options are inhibited and the person acts. All of this can happen very rapidly, within the span of a few minutes or even seconds. People who attempt suicide tend to be sensitive to negative interpersonal situations and experiences but are less sensitive or "immune" to positive interpersonal situations and experiences. This imbalance can lead them to act upon negative emotions and expectations that have not been sufficiently modulated by positive emotions and expectations. Strengthening an individual's responsivity to positive experiences while decreasing their reactivity to negative experiences could serve as a braking system that prevents the emergence of suicidal behaviors. This is exactly what the strategies used in CPT and BCBT are designed to do. These treatments may "undo" or reverse the difficulties in planning ahead, generating options, and controlling emotions and impulses that many suicidal individuals experience; instead, enhancing their ability to experience positive emotions and to expect positive outcomes in the future. When Jenny completed CPT, she had improved enough that she no longer met the diagnostic criteria for PTSD. She also felt that suicide could be left behind; she had come to realize that there were other ways to respond to stressful situations in life and to think about the trauma that had haunted her for so long.

If we had taken MRI scans of Jenny's brain, we may have seen changes within her central executive network along the lines of what Abdallah found in his study of patients with PTSD who completed CPT. We also might have seen changes in her default mode network; the increase in positive emotions described by Jenny may have been reflected by increased activation of the ventromedial prefrontal cortex during stressful situations, implicating a buffering effect of approach-related emotions on withdrawal-related emotions. As Jenny explained, approach-related emotions like happiness and joy did not eliminate problems or stressful situations and did not negate the experience of withdrawal-related emotions like anxiety, depression, and guilt, but they did help to put withdrawal-related emotions in check, thereby reducing their impact on decision-making processes.

Six months after finishing treatment, Jenny called to let us know how she was doing. She said that she was doing very well and was no longer experiencing the unwanted thoughts and memories, self-blame, and guilt about her sexual assault. She felt as though she was finally in control of her emotions again and was experiencing positive emotions like happiness and joy on a regular basis. Jenny also reported another important change: She was no longer regularly thinking about suicide. "I can have a good life," she explained. "I realize now that I can be happy—truly happy—not just fake happy." Unfortunately, many of the people in her life—family, friends, and coworkers—didn't share her newfound zest for life. Just as they had been unsupportive in the aftermath of her rape, these individuals were unsupportive now. Jenny had changed, of course, but no one else had. Instead of celebrating her accomplishments, they were skeptical that any change had occurred at all, and they continued to treat her as though she were, in Jenny's words, "damaged goods." She had learned important skills in treatment that provided considerable benefit, but her environment had not changed, and the hazards that threatened her well-being remained present.

For Jenny, returning home from treatment was like visiting Chernobyl with a hazmat suit. The hazmat suit offers protection, but if the suit ever rips or frays, or is misaligned slightly, she could be exposed to dangerous levels of radiation and harmed as a result. Wearing a hazmat suit affords some protection when visiting Chernobyl, but if you stay long enough, radiation exposure and its harmful consequences are inevitable. Unfortunately, the radiation contamination cannot be removed. Staying away from Chernobyl is therefore the safest option. In like fashion, Jenny decided that it was best for her to enact an engineering control by removing herself from the family, friends, and coworkers who served as a hazard to her well-being. "I'm moving away from home because I want to start a new chapter in my life," she explained. "People here still see me as the old Jenny. I thought they would eventually change once I had changed, but they haven't. It's time to leave that behind. It's time to be happy again." Jenny had moved many times before to escape stressful and psychologically hazardous environments, but this time around she also was motivated by the desire to seek out positive experiences and environments that could promote and support her well-being.

Mental health treatment can help individuals create meaningful and satisfying lives, but it's not the *only* way to achieve this outcome; our environments also have an incredibly profound effect on our well-being. Indeed, the environment probably plays a much bigger role than we assume. Consider, for example, the results of two studies we conducted examining how group membership can protect people from the emotional consequences of stress exposure and reduce the probability of thinking about suicide. In this study, we asked 997 military personnel who were assigned to 40 different units to fill out a survey asking them about how often they experienced positive emotions like happiness and joy, how often and intensely they experienced symptoms of depression and PTSD, what kinds of stressful events they had experienced during their lives, how much support they received from other people, and if they had recently thought about death or suicide. Some of our findings were not particularly surprising: Service members who said they were happier also tended to report less severe symptoms of PTSD, for example. The more interesting findings indicated that the emotional state and perceptions of available support had a stronger correlation with a service member's psychological stress and suicidal thinking than the service member's own ratings of their emotional state and available support, suggesting that service members benefited more from being around people who were happier and felt highly supported than they did from their own happiness and perceived level of support.

Promoting positive emotional states and ensuring the availability of support across groups—whether these groups be military units, neighborhoods, faith communities, social clubs, workplaces, cities, or regions—can reduce each individual group member's risk for attempting suicide even when an individual is not experiencing these positive emotions and feels unsupported themselves, akin to how being surrounded by cars equipped with lane departure and blind spot warning systems can reduce our risk for collision even if our own car lacks these safety features. If, for example, you and I are driving next to each other on the highway and you start to drift into my lane, but stop when your alert system warns you, I have personally benefited from your car's lane departure alert system even though I do not have this same safety feature in my car. When many cars have these safety features, the probability that *anyone* will get into an accident drops because all of us are benefiting from the accumulated protection of the many cars that possess these features. Each driver benefits from the safety features of their own car, but they benefit to a much larger degree from the safety features of everyone else sharing the road with them. Positive emotional states, which can be "transferred" from one person to another within social groups, probably work in a similar way: They help us to self-correct when we start to drift off course, but even if we are not experiencing positive emotions ourselves, we nonetheless benefit from regularly interacting with others who do. Context matters.

Jenny's case also highlights another important lesson: Suicide prevention cannot just be about getting rid of pain and discomfort and life problems, it must also be about creating positive experiences and strengthening quality of life. To do suicide prevention well, we have to do more than just stop people from dying—we also have to make life worth living.

Creating Lives Worth Living

This is one of the key lessons that I learned during our first BCBT study. In that study, we asked patients to share their impressions of the treatment they had received, whether BCBT or status quo treatment. For example, we asked them what they liked best about their treatment, what they liked least, what they thought was most helpful, what they thought we should change, and so on. We quickly identified a trend among those who had received BCBT: These patients were reporting improvements in all sorts of symptoms of mental illness, such as depression, anxiety, suicidal thoughts, and sleep problems, but this wasn't what they found to be most helpful about the treatment. Over and over again, patients were telling us the treatment was most helpful because it improved "good" things, such as happiness, hope, purpose, and self-efficacy. They were more hopeful about life, believed that things were going to be OK after all, and had a sense of purpose. When bad things happened in life, they also felt like they knew how to respond more effectively instead of "losing my cool," as one patient explained. "Life is full of bad things happening," another patient noted, "but you can always look forward and try to make the best of the future." Some of the people who received status quo treatment reported similar benefits, but not to the same extent or degree as those who received the suicide-focused treatment. Like Jenny, they were seeing themselves from a different perspective. Also like Jenny, their quality of life had improved.

We also found differences with respect to how our patients' wish to live changed over time. We assessed their wish to live separately from their wish to die because we suspected that the wish to live and the wish to die were not opposite ends of a pole. When someone has a strong wish to live, they often also have a low wish to die, but not always; sometimes people want to die, but they also want to live. Overall, we found that the wish to live—but not the wish to die—distinguished those individuals who made a suicide attempt during or soon after treatment. We also found some evidence that a stronger wish to live inhibited or blocked the emergence of suicidal behavior, even among those who possessed a strong wish to die. A weaker wish to die did not inhibit the emergence of suicidal behavior, however, suggesting that positive rather than negative psychological states and experiences played an especially important preventative role. Patients who received BCBT appeared to be better at activating or increasing their wish to live in a protective manner, essentially counteracting and (ultimately) destabilizing their wish to die. These patients continued to experience stressful situations in life, but they had acquired the capacity to inhibit their initial reactions to these situations, to consider alternative responses, and to select other goal-directed behaviors. In the end, their probability of attempting suicide was reduced because they were seeing the world in a different way and making different decisions when faced with uncertainty and under duress. They weren't just taking their foot off the accelerator to avoid a collision, they were also pressing the brake.

Finding reasons for living

Another central feature of our patients' new decision-making style when in crisis involved the ability to remember and explicitly consider their reasons for living. Reasons for living reflect those aspects of one's life that motivate the wish to live; if you have a reason to live, you are much less likely to make decisions that threaten this motive. Marsha Linehan recognized this fact over three decades ago when she was developing dialectical behavior therapy (DBT), the first psychological treatment to consistently demonstrate an ability to reduce suicidal behaviors. Consistent with this perspective, a central tenet of DBT is to help individuals create lives worth living; this same tenet has since been preserved within BCBT and the crisis response plan (CRP). In BCBT, for instance, we spend an entire session talking about these reasons for living and then write these reasons for living on an index card. Patients are directed to carry the card around as a constant reminder of the positive things they have in life, and to read the index card on a regular basis, even when *not* emotionally upset. This strategy essentially teaches suicidal individuals how to remember what is good and meaningful about their lives and helps them to build and expand these parts of their lives.

In our study, we found that a good number of patients who visited our offices months after finishing treatment were still carrying their reasons-for-living card in their pockets. Others didn't carry their card with them but told us that they had decorated their card and hung it up on their refrigerator so they could see it every day. Still others described additional strategies or techniques for reminding themselves of their reasons for living. Perhaps even more surprising was hearing from some patients about how they had shared their reasons-for-living card with a friend or acquaintance in crisis, explaining how it helped them to keep perspective during tough times. These patients didn't just tell their friends about the card, though; in many cases, they would help their friends to create a card of their own, thereby transferring the benefits of their own positive emotional states to others.

Because reasons for living seemed to play such an important role in overcoming suicidal thoughts and reducing the probability of suicidal behaviors, we subsequently integrated reasons for living into the CRP by asking acutely suicidal individuals in the midst of an emotional crisis to spend some time thinking about their reasons for living or for not killing themselves. This was, understandably, very difficult for many people to do while in crisis; "I don't have any reasons" was a common response. We found that one of the most effective ways to help people who felt they had no reasons for living was to approach this situation like a lost set of keys. Most of us have lost our keys at some point and experienced the frustration and despair that often comes with this situation. Being unable to find our keys is not the same as our keys ceasing to exist, however. Those keys were *somewhere*, and we probably used one or more of the following strategies to find them: thinking of where we were and what we doing when we last had them, retracing our steps, and asking others for help. Reasons for living, we explained, were the same. Sometimes we can't find them but that doesn't mean they don't exist, and we can use some of these same strategies to find them: thinking about what we were doing when we last felt that we had reasons for living, retracing our steps in life to revisit times and places when we had reasons for living, and asking others to help us find them. Just as we may not have found our lost keys right away, we also may not find our lost reasons for living right away, but if we remind ourselves that they must exist somewhere, we may be able to keep up the search long enough to find them again.

I've used this technique many, many times with suicidal patients and found it to be especially powerful and useful, even though it can sometimes be a very difficult process. With help and support, however, we have found that most suicidal people are eventually able to identify at least one reason for living, at which point we would ask them to tell us a story about that reason. We elicited these stories about their reasons for living in an attempt to strengthen activation of the default mode network, the system of our brain that is involved in accessing and reflecting upon specific memories from our lives. Suicidal individuals struggle to access the details of these types of memories, resulting in overgeneralized or nonspecific memories. If you ask someone in a suicidal crisis to describe a social event they recently attended, for example, they might respond with an answer along the lines of "a party." If you were to ask that same question of someone who is not suicidal and has never attempted suicide, you would probably receive a more detailed response; something like, "I went to a party two weeks ago at my friend Jon's house." They also might tell a story about a particular noteworthy detail from the night.

Strengthening an individual's ability to remember specific memories from their life, especially memories that elicit positive emotions, could increase activation and interconnectivity within the default mode network, thereby making this information available to the central executive network when engaged in the tasks of identifying and selecting behavioral responses to a stressful situation. We have yet to conduct studies to know if this is what *actually* happens when a suicidal individual is asked to think about their reasons for living, but we do know that this strategy significantly increases positive emotions and optimism among acutely suicidal individuals and results in larger reductions in their urge to act upon their suicidal impulses. More recently, we've also found that the positive emotional states lead to faster reductions in suicidal thinking among acutely suicidal patients after they reflect upon and share stories about their reasons for living. In the midst of a suicidal crisis, taking a few minutes to reflect upon what makes life worth living can help someone find their internal braking system and slow down.

Some reasons for living are more powerful than others

In my own experience, the most common reasons for living involve things such as family members, friends, pets, and aspirations for the future. These general categories overlap with several categories of reasons for living identified by Linehan several decades ago when she and her collaborators developed a questionnaire they named the *Reasons for Living Inventory*. Early research using this scale identified six categories of reasons for living: survival and coping beliefs, responsibility to family, child-related concerns, fear of suicide, fear of social disapproval, and moral objections to suicide (see Table 8.1). Of these six categories, the first four were much stronger among individuals who had never been suicidal or had relatively mild suicidal thoughts as compared to individuals who had been severely suicidal or attempted

Table 8.1 Categories of Reasons for Living Assessed by the *Reasons for Living Inventory*

Category	Definition
Survival and Coping Beliefs	The desire to overcome hardship and a generally optimistic perspective about oneself and the problems one faces
Responsibility to Family	A sense of duty and commitment to one's family, and concern that one's death could negatively impact one's family
Child-Related Concerns	Worrying about the safety and well-being of one's children
Fear of Suicide	Anxiety and uncertainty about death
Fear of Social Disapproval	Worries that one would be negatively judged and evaluated by others
Moral Objections to Suicide	Social and/or spiritual beliefs or proscriptions against suicide

suicide in the past. The last two categories, however, fear of social disapproval and moral objections to suicide, were not as useful for distinguishing those who had previously been suicidal or attempted suicide.

The Reasons for Living Inventory and several shortened versions of this scale have since been used in research studies with many different types of individuals, including adolescents, adults receiving mental health treatment, and prison inmates. Across studies, individuals who score higher on the Reasons for Living Inventory are generally less likely to have attempted suicide and report less intense suicidal thoughts. I've even used a shortened version of the scale in my own research. In one of our studies, for instance, we found that military personnel who scored higher on the survival and coping beliefs and responsibility to family subscales also reported less severe suicidal ideation and emotional distress, and described their lives as more meaningful and full of purpose. Higher scores on the responsibility to family category were also associated with reduced risk for suicide attempts during the next six months; being concerned about the welfare of one's family seemed to reduce the probability of suicidal behavior.

Other researchers also have found that the survival and coping beliefs and responsibility to family categories have the strongest associations with suicidal thoughts and behaviors. These are interesting findings to me for at least two reasons. First, although responsibility to family differentiated those who would attempt suicide within the next six months, it did not differentiate those who had *previously* attempted suicide. Something that was correlated with a decreased probability of *future* suicide attempts was not correlated with the probability of a *past* suicide attempt. Second, although survival and coping beliefs had a stronger correlation than responsibility to family with recent suicidal *thinking*, responsibility to family had a stronger correlation than survival and coping beliefs with suicidal *behaviors*, suggesting that things in our lives that reduce the likelihood that we will try to kill ourselves may not be the same things in our lives that modulate our thoughts about suicide.

What is it about survival and coping beliefs and responsibility to family that helps to reduce suicidal thoughts and behaviors to a greater degree than the other categories? Examining the specific items that make up these two scales may provide some clues. I've therefore listed in Box 8.1 the 14 items used in the *Brief Reasons for Living Inventory*—the version of the scale used

---

Box 8.1 *Brief Reasons for Living Inventory* Items Used to Assess Each Reason for Living Category

Item

Fear of Social Disapproval

    I am concerned about what others would think of me

    Other people would think I am weak and selfish

    I would not want people to think I did not have control over my life

Moral Objections

    I believe only God has the right to end a life

    My religious beliefs forbid it

    I consider it morally wrong

Survival and Coping Beliefs

    I believe I can find other solutions to my problems

    I believe everything has a way of working out for the best

    I have the courage to face life

Responsibility to Family

    My family depends upon me and needs me

    I love and enjoy my family too much and could not leave them

    It would hurt my family too much and I would not want them to suffer

Fear of Suicide

    I am afraid of death

    I am afraid of the unknown

in my research study. These items also are used in the full Reasons for Living Inventory originally developed by Linehan, so they provide a reasonable picture of each category. Reading through this list, the items that make up the survival and coping beliefs and responsibility to family categories appear to differ from the remaining three categories in one important way: The language used in these items asks about positive psychological and emotional states. The survival and coping beliefs items, for instance, assess hope (*I believe I can find other solutions to my problems*), self-confidence (*I have the courage to face life*), and optimism (*I believe everything has a way of working out for the best*), and the responsibility to family items ask about purpose and meaning (*My family depends upon me and needs me*), love and happiness (*I love and enjoy my family too much and could not leave them*), and compassion (*It would hurt my family too much and I would not want them to suffer*). The items used to assess the fear of social disapproval, moral objections, and fear of suicide categories, by comparison, assess the desire to avoid negative emotional states such as anxiety (*I am concerned about what others would think about me*), shame (*I consider it morally wrong*), and fear (*I am afraid of death*).

Reasons for living that are motivated by the desire to generate or experience positive emotional states may, therefore, be better at offsetting suicidal thoughts and reducing the probability of suicidal behaviors than reasons for living that are motivated by the desire to avoid or withdraw from uncomfortable situations and negative emotional states. Interestingly, the desire to avoid or withdraw from negative emotional states is known to be an especially strong motivator of suicidal behavior. Fear of social disapproval, moral objections, and fear of suicide involve a similar psychological process: avoidance of negative psychological states. Survival and coping beliefs and responsibility to family, in contrast, involve approach-related psychological processes that contradict the avoidance-related processes that drive suicidal behavior. Approach-related reasons for living may be especially potent as an internal braking system when experiencing an emotional crisis.

It's important to note that remembering your reasons for living and experiencing positive emotional states doesn't mean your life is completely absent of problems, stress, or symptoms of mental illness. Reasons for living and positive emotional states can put these things into perspective, however. They provide balance, enabling us to remember or rediscover a sense of purpose and meaning. For some, reasons for living and positive emotional states can provide an opportunity to create a new sense of purpose and meaning that didn't exist before. In the midst of a suicidal crisis, many individuals question the purpose of living, finding it hard to remember their reasons for living and what gives their lives a sense of meaning. Over time, the majority of suicidal individuals come to realize that they really *do* have purpose and meaning and reasons for living, even though they also may have problems that still need to be solved, face challenges that can seem insurmountable, and experience painful emotions.

Consider, for example, a survey we recently conducted in which we asked 997 people how frequently they experienced positive emotions such as happiness and joy, the extent to which they perceived that their lives were filled with meaning, and when they had last thought about suicide (we provided the following options: within the past week, the past month, the past year, or more than one year ago). We decided to study happiness and meaning in life because these two concepts are considered central components of well-being. Our results showed that happiness and meaning in life scores generally increased as the time since the most recent suicidal thought extended further into the past; people who had been suicidal more than year prior were happier on average than people who had been suicidal in the past year; people who had been suicidal more than one month ago were happier on average than people who had been suicidal within the past week, and so on.

Our results also suggested that it doesn't take very long for a previously suicidal individual to report an average to above average sense of happiness and meaning in life. Among those who were currently suicidal, for instance, only 25 out of 100 reported average or above average happiness and 37 out of 100 reported average or above average meaning in life. Among those who had not thought about suicide for at least one month, however, these numbers doubled: 55 out of 100 reported average or above average happiness and 63 out of 100 reported average or above average meaning in life. These numbers were even higher among those who had not thought about suicide for at least one year: 76 out of 100 reported average or above average happiness and 80 out of 100 reported average or above average meaning in life.

Not everyone experiences these improvements at the same rate, of course, but these results suggest there is a better than 50–50 chance that someone who is currently thinking about suicide will report an average level of well-being within a few months.

Overcoming suicidal thoughts and living a meaningful, high-quality life is quite likely, even for individuals who never access mental health treatment. When overcome by suicidal despair, however, it doesn't seem as though things will ever get better and it doesn't seem as though we'll be able to endure long enough for things to get better. One factor that contributes to this perception is uncertainty; we don't know when things will actually get better or how long we'll feel this way, so the wait seems unbearable. Having a sense of purpose and meaning, and/or being able to remember one's reasons for living, both of which contribute to positive emotional states, may help to counteract these perceptions. Although positive emotional states do not necessarily eliminate negative emotions, research suggests they support perspective-taking and planning for the future, and help us to identify and use adaptive coping strategies. Positive emotional states may therefore "undo" the harmful effects of negative emotions such as cognitive rigidity, cognitive bias, and avoidance, all of which increase vulnerability to suicidal behavior. When we experience positive emotions and know our reasons for living, waiting for the second marshmallow instead of eating the one marshmallow in front of us becomes easier.

Suicide Prevention Requires Much More than Treatment

As Jenny's story shows, positive emotional states, quality of life, and the wish to live can be promoted via mental health treatment, but they also can be influenced by our environments. Taking steps to create environments that can promote positive emotions and quality of life would enable us to foster the conditions that are best suited for the purposes of suicide prevention. More importantly, an environmentally focused prevention-by-design approach would help us to address the many social and psychological hazards that can increase the risk for suicidal behaviors but cannot be remedied with mental health treatment: underemployment, financial insecurity, discrimination, lack of health insurance, and more. Establishing a meaningful life is possible—even likely—but it's much harder to achieve when you live in an environment or community that lacks institutions, programs, and resources that promote a high quality of life. This is the conundrum that Jenny, and so many others like her, faced. Jenny decided to relocate and "start over" because she determined that it was "time to be happy again," but not everyone has the resources available to pursue this same course for themselves. They may have changed—or desire to change—but their environment gets in the way of establishing a life worth living.

Broadening our perspective beyond the suicidal individual with their presumed mental illness is the final way that we can become productively stupid about suicide. Changing our environment in ways that strengthen or promote reasons for living and subjective well-being can influence the probability of suicidal behaviors (see Box 8.2). These factors may not have an especially large effect on suicide, but as we discussed in an earlier chapter, when it comes to something like suicide, small things can carry disproportionate weight, and the slightest of nudges can determine on which side of the tipping point someone falls. The challenge we face, of course, is that none of the social factors that promote well-being can be controlled by any of us individually; they can only be influenced by groups of individuals. Creating lives worth living requires the collective effort of many people working together and sharing a sense of responsibility. Governmental bodies can, for instance, enhance well-being through legislative action and policies designed to strengthen social services such as unemployment protection and access to health care, and through zoning laws and urban development plans designed to promote social connections and increase positive emotional states (e.g., access to green spaces, reduced commute time). Corporations and businesses can enhance well-being by working to reduce pay inequities, strengthening pensions, providing better healthcare coverage plans, and promoting expressions of appreciation, gratitude, and respect. Expressions of gratitude and respect also have been shown to promote well-being and reduce suicidal thinking by promoting optimism and meaning in life while also reducing

---

Box 8.2. Strategies that Could Prevent Suicide by Improving Well-Being and Quality of Life

1. Enhance financial security through increased wages and improved retirement benefits
2. Improve the health and attractiveness of natural environments (e.g., less pollution)
3. Expand access to healthcare services
4. Improve the affordability of healthcare services
5. Design neighborhoods and communities that facilitate social connections (e.g., easy access to parks and green space)
6. Support and encourage expressions of gratitude and appreciation within social groups

hopelessness; such expressions are important within families and other social groups including faith communities, schools, and social clubs.

Each of these strategies could reduce the probability of suicidal behaviors
through a combination of their direct impact upon each of us and, owing
to the transfer of positive emotions and well-being that occurs within social groups, their indirect impact through all the people who surround us.
A rising tide lifts all boats. If we are surrounded by things that improve our
quality of life, we can reduce the probability of suicidal behavior and facilitate the creation of postsuicidal lives by strengthening the value of living.
This is, to me, the true heart and soul of the oft-cited mantra *suicide prevention is everyone's business.* Suicide prevention being everyone's business
doesn't mean that everyone needs to be conducting suicide risk screenings
and repeatedly imploring people to pursue mental health treatment. Rather,
it means that we should be working together on a daily basis to create lives
worth living.

Notes

Introduction

1. Also known as LSA Anaconda and Balad Air Base.
2. Trauma center levels are designated by roman numerals ranging from I (highest severity) to V (lowest severity). These designations refer to the kinds of resources available at the facility and the number of patients treated on an annual basis. Level I trauma centers provide comprehensive care for every aspect of an injury, have 24-hour coverage by general surgeons and other surgical and medical specialties, and serve as a referral resource for other facilities located nearby. During Operation Iraqi Freedom, the Air Force Theater Hospital was one of the largest and most advanced hospitals in Iraq.
3. Medical transport flights required a balancing of medical risk and operational risk. If the patient's medical condition was dire or very severe, transport flights would be scheduled despite worse flying conditions. If a patient's medical condition was not severe, however, transport flights would be delayed until flying conditions were less risky. Because there is no potential for clinical worsening for deceased individuals, medical risk did not outweigh the risks associated with the flight itself.

Chapter 1

1. The military has a much larger percentage of men and young adults than the U.S. general population: approximately 85% of military personnel versus 49% of the U.S. general population are men, and approximately 67% of military personnel versus 42% of the U.S. general population are younger than 30 years. Because suicide rates differ across gender and age groups, adjustments are typically made when comparing military and general population rates to reduce bias arising from these very different demographic profiles.
2. Here, I am only focusing on adults. The total number of U.S. suicides in 2017, including both adults and children, was actually 47,173.
3. Several years later, after moving to Utah, I learned of another close connection to Pete: The wife of an undergraduate student who volunteered in my research lab was one of the enlisted technicians who worked alongside Pete while they were deployed to Iraq.

Chapter 2

1. In the U.S. Air Force, a "First Shirt"—often referred to simply as "the Shirt"—is a colloquial term for the First Sergeant, a special duty held by a senior noncommissioned officer. The primary duty of the First Sergeant is to support morale and welfare and to promote good conduct among enlisted personnel. In this role, First Sergeants often intervene with or assist enlisted personnel in need.
2. The confidence interval provides an estimate of a particular finding's precision. If a confidence interval is very wide, then we can conclude that our finding is not very precise. Conversely, if a confidence interval is narrow, we have more confidence about the finding's precision.
3. As mentioned earlier, the estimated annual prevalence rate of mental illness in the United States is 26%, placing us at the upper end of this range.

Chapter 3

1. If you have visited a primary care or family medicine practitioner in the past few years, it's quite likely that you have completed this screening tool yourself.
2. In order to increase confidence in the anonymity of this third tool, military personnel were directed to seal their responses in an unmarked envelope and then deposit the envelope in an unmarked box that was kept separate from all the other surveys and information.

Chapter 4

1. Preparatory behaviors include actions taken to prepare for one's death or for making a suicide attempt, such as writing a suicide note, acquiring the materials needed to make the attempt (e.g., collecting pills, purchasing a firearm), and/or reducing the probability that someone will intervene. Rehearsal behaviors include practicing a suicide attempt or engaging in a "dry run."
2. This provides further evidence contradicting the traditional perspective that suicide results from or is caused by mental illness. If mental illness caused suicide, we would expect that various indicators of mental illness such as depression, anxiety, and hopelessness would distinguish between low suicide risk and high suicide risk states.

Chapter 5

1. If, by chance, you are interested in reading some of these works yourself, you can access many from the book's only digital archive, available at https://ethicsofsuicide.lib.utah.edu.

Chapter 6

1. Here, I use the term cognitive behavioral therapy for suicide prevention (CBT-SP) inclusively to refer to two separate but similar treatment protocols: cognitive therapy for suicide prevention (CT-SP) and brief cognitive behavioral therapy for suicide prevention (BCBT).

2. Another iteration of the CRP is called the safety planning intervention, which was described by Barbara Stanley and Greg Brown in a 2012 publication. The safety planning intervention contains many of the same components as CRP, but uses a form instead of an index card.

3. In a new study currently underway, we are investigating this possibility by comparing BCBT to present-centered therapy, a type of mental health treatment that has been shown to reduce the symptoms of mental illness and suicidal thinking. In addition to comparing rates of suicidal behaviors among patients receiving each treatment, we also will examine how the two treatments impact decision-making style. If decision-making processes truly are involved in reducing the probability of suicidal behaviors, we would expect to see significant differences in decision-making style *and* suicidal behaviors between the two treatments.

4. The Bernecker study used data from the first treatment study comparing BCBT to status quo treatment that Rudd and I completed with the U.S. Army. On the whole, military personnel tend to use more lethal methods when attempting suicide than civilians; as a result, suicidal behavior among military personnel is much more likely to result in death. In several simulations, Bernecker consequently used CDC data to estimate the treatment's effects on suicide death under these more conservative conditions; the values presented here are those conservative estimates to maximize their relevance to all suicides.

Chapter 8

1. Names and details of this story have been changed to protect the privacy of the individuals involved.

2. The other recommended treatments are prolonged exposure therapy (PE) and eye movement desensitization and reprocessing (EMDR).

3. The reductions in suicidal ideation observed now in multiple studies of CPT, as well as other trauma-focused therapies such as PE, stand in sharp contrast to the still widespread myth among mental health professionals that these therapies are unsafe for trauma survivors who are suicidal. A small number of trauma survivors do experience an increase in suicidal thoughts during trauma-focused therapies, but so do trauma survivors who receive other types of mental health treatment. Finding new ways to efficiently reduce suicide risk and PTSD symptom severity among high-risk trauma survivors is a central focus of several studies currently underway.

Bibliography

Introduction

1. Ellenberg, J. (2015). *How Not to Be Wrong: The Power of Mathematical Thinking.* New York: Penguin Press.
2. Nye, L. (2019, March 27). *The Mathematician Who Saved Hundreds of Flight Crews.* Retrieved from https://www.wearethemighty.com/history/abraham-wald-survivor-bias-ww2
3. Rittel, H. W. J., & Webber, M. M. (1973). Dilemmas in a general theory of planning. *Policy Sciences, 4,* 155–169.
4. Knapp, R. (2008). Wholesome design or wicked problems. *Public Sphere Project.* Retrieved from http://publicsphereproject.org/content/wholesome-design-wicked-problems
5. Rich, J. (2009). Where death delights to serve the living. *HEAL: Humanism Evolving Through Arts and Literature, 1,* 69.

Chapter 1

1. Defense Suicide Prevention Office (n.d.). *Defense Suicide Prevention Office.* Retrieved from https://www.dspo.mil/Prevention/Data-Surveillance/DoDSER-Annual-Reports
2. Joiner, T. E. (2007). *Why People Die by Suicide.* Cambridge, MA: Harvard University Press.
3. Substance Abuse and Mental Health Service Administration. (2018). *Key Substance Use and Mental Health Indicators in the United States: Results from the 2017 National Survey on Drug Use and Health (HHS Publication No. SMA 18-5068, NSDUH Series H-53).* Rockville, MD: Center for Behavioral Health Statistics and Quality, Substance Abuse and Mental Health Services Administration.
4. Bryan, C. J., Morrow, C. E., Anestis, M. D., & Joiner, T. E. (2010). A preliminary test of the interpersonal-psychological theory of suicidal behavior in a military sample. *Personality and Individual Differences, 48,* 347–350.
5. Van Orden, K. A., Witte, T. K., Gordon, K. H., Bender, T. W., & Joiner Jr, T. E. (2008). Suicidal desire and the capability for suicide: Tests of the interpersonal-psychological theory of suicidal behavior among adults. *Journal of Consulting and Clinical Psychology, 76,* 72–83.
6. Boisseau, C. L., Yen, S., Markowitz, J. C., Grilo, C. M., Sanislow, C. A., Shea, M. T., ... & McGlashan, T. H. (2013). Individuals with single versus multiple suicide attempts over 10 years of prospective follow-up. *Comprehensive Psychiatry, 54,* 238–242.

7. Bryan, C. J., Clemans, T. A., & Hernandez, A. M. (2012). Perceived burdensomeness, fearlessness of death, and suicidality among deployed military personnel. *Personality and Individual Differences, 52*, 374–379.

8. Bryan, C. J., Cukrowicz, K. C., West, C. L., & Morrow, C. E. (2010). Combat experience and the acquired capability for suicide. *Journal of Clinical Psychology, 66*, 1044–1056.

9. Bryan, C. J., & Cukrowicz, K. C. (2011). Associations between types of combat violence and the acquired capability for suicide. *Suicide and Life-Threatening Behavior, 41*, 126–136.

10. Department of the Army. (2010). *Army Health Promotion, Risk Reduction, Suicide Prevention Report 2010*. Washington, DC: Department of the Army.

11. LeardMann, C. A., Powell, T. M., Smith, T. C., Bell, M. R., Smith, B., Boyko, E. J., . . . & Hoge, C. W. (2013). Risk factors associated with suicide in current and former US military personnel. *JAMA, 310*, 496–506.

12. Schoenbaum, M., Kessler, R. C., Gilman, S. E., Colpe, L. J., Heeringa, S. G., Stein, M. B., . . . & Cox, K. L. (2014). Predictors of suicide and accident death in the Army Study to Assess Risk and Resilience in Servicemembers (Army STARRS): Results from the Army Study to Assess Risk and Resilience in Servicemembers (Army STARRS). *JAMA Psychiatry, 71*, 493–503.

13. Reger, M. A., Smolenski, D. J., Skopp, N. A., Metzger-Abamukang, M. J., Kang, H. K., Bullman, T. A., . . . & Gahm, G. A. (2015). Risk of suicide among US military service members following Operation Enduring Freedom or Operation Iraqi Freedom deployment and separation from the US military. *JAMA Psychiatry, 72*, 561–569.

14. Nock, M. K., Stein, M. B., Heeringa, S. G., Ursano, R. J., Colpe, L. J., Fullerton, C. S., . . . & Zaslavsky, A. M. (2014). Prevalence and correlates of suicidal behavior among soldiers: Results from the Army Study to Assess Risk and Resilience in Servicemembers (Army STARRS). *JAMA Psychiatry, 71*, 514–522.

15. Maguen, S., Metzler, T. J., Bosch, J., Marmar, C. R., Knight, S. J., & Neylan, T. C. (2012). Killing in combat may be independently associated with suicidal ideation. *Depression and Anxiety, 29*, 918–923.

16. Maguen, S., Luxton, D. D., Skopp, N. A., Gahm, G. A., Reger, M. A., Metzler, T. J., & Marmar, C. R. (2011). Killing in combat, mental health symptoms, and suicidal ideation in Iraq war veterans. *Journal of Anxiety Disorders, 25*, 563–567.

17. Bryan, C. J., McNaughton-Cassill, M., & Osman, A. (2013). Age and belongingness moderate the effects of combat exposure on suicidal ideation among active duty Air Force personnel. *Journal of Affective Disorders, 150*, 1226–1229.

18. Bryan, C. J., Griffith, J. E., Pace, B. T., Hinkson, K., Bryan, A. O., Clemans, T. A., & Imel, Z. E. (2015). Combat exposure and risk for suicidal thoughts and behaviors among military personnel and veterans: A systematic review and meta-analysis. *Suicide and Life-Threatening Behavior, 45*, 633–649.

19. Stone, D. M., Simon, T. R., Fowler, K. A., Kegler, S. R., Yuan, K., Holland, K. M., & Crosby, A. E. (2018). Vital Signs: Trends in state suicide rates—United States, 1999–2016 and circumstances contributing to suicide—27 states, 2015. *Morbidity and Mortality Weekly Report, 67*, 617–624.

20. World Health Organization. (2018). *Suicide rate estimates, age-standardized: Estimates by country*. Retrieved from http://apps.who.int/gho/data/node.main. MHSUICIDEASDR?lang=en

21. Williams, S. S. (2016). The terrorist inside my husband's brain. *Neurology, 87*, 1308–1311.

Chapter 2

1. Centers for Disease Control and Prevention. (n.d.). *Web-Based Injury Statistics Query and Reporting System (WISQARS) Fatal Injury Data*. Retrieved from https://www. cdc.gov/injury/wisqars.fatal.html
2. Franklin, J. C., Ribeiro, J. D., Fox, K. R., Bentley, K. H., Kleiman, E. M., Huang, X., . . . & Nock, M. K. (2017). Risk factors for suicidal thoughts and behaviors: A meta-analysis of 50 years of research. *Psychological Bulletin, 143*, 187–232.
3. United States Census Bureau (2018). *QuickFacts United States*. Retrieved from https://www.census.gov/quickfacts/fact/table/US/PST045218
4. Kessler, R. C., Chiu, W. T., Demler, O., & Walters, E. E. (2005). Prevalence, severity, and comorbidity of 12-month DSM-IV disorders in the National Comorbidity Survey Replication. *Archives of General Psychiatry, 62*, 617–627.
5. Linehan, M. M., Comtois, K. A., Murray, A. M., Brown, M. Z., Gallop, R. J., Heard, H. L., . . . & Lindenboim, N. (2006). Two-year randomized controlled trial and follow-up of dialectical behavior therapy vs therapy by experts for suicidal behaviors and borderline personality disorder. *Archives of General Psychiatry, 63*, 757–766.
6. Brown, G. K., Ten Have, T., Henriques, G. R., Xie, S. X., Hollander, J. E., & Beck, A. T. (2005). Cognitive therapy for the prevention of suicide attempts: A randomized controlled trial. *JAMA, 294*, 563–570.
7. Rudd, M. D., Bryan, C. J., Wertenberger, E. G., Peterson, A. L., Young-McCaughan, S., Mintz, J., . . . & Wilkinson, E. (2015). Brief cognitive-behavioral therapy effects on post-treatment suicide attempts in a military sample: Results of a randomized clinical trial with 2-year follow-up. *American Journal of Psychiatry, 172*, 441–449.
8. American Psychiatric Association (2013). *Diagnostic and Statistical Manual of Mental Disorders (DSM-5)*. Washington, DC: American Psychiatric Publications.
9. Carta, M. G., Balestrieri, M., Murru, A., & Hardoy, M. C. (2009). Adjustment Disorder: Epidemiology, diagnosis and treatment. *Clinical Practice and Epidemiology in Mental Health, 5*, 15.
10. Evans, S. C., Reed, G. M., Roberts, M. C., Esparza, P., Watts, A. D., Correia, J. M., . . . & Saxena, S. (2013). Psychologists' perspectives on the diagnostic classification of mental disorders: Results from the WHO-IUPsyS Global Survey. *International Journal of Psychology, 48*, 177–193.
11. Casey, P., Dowrick, C., & Wilkinson, G. (2001). Adjustment disorders: Fault line in the psychiatric glossary. *The British Journal of Psychiatry, 179*, 479–481.
12. Cavanagh, J. T., Carson, A. J., Sharpe, M., & Lawrie, S. M. (2003). Psychological autopsy studies of suicide: a systematic review. *Psychological Medicine, 33*, 395–405.
13. Berman, A. (2006). The other 10 percent. *Newslink, 33*, 3.
14. Hjelmeland, H., Dieserud, G., Dyregrov, K., Knizek, B. L., & Leenaars, A. A. (2012). Psychological autopsy studies as diagnostic tools: Are they methodologically flawed? *Death Studies, 36*, 605–626.

Chapter 3

1. Cavanaugh, J. T., Carson, A. J., Sharpe, M., & Lawrie, S. M. (2003). Psychological autopsy studies of suicide: A systematic review. *Psychological Medicine, 33*, 395–405.
2. Centers for Disease Control and Prevention. (n.d.). *Web-Based Injury Statistics Query and Reporting System (WISQARS) Fatal Injury Data*. Retrieved from https://www. cdc.gov/injury/wisqars.fatal.html

3. DeVon, H. A., Rosenfeld, A., Steffen, A. D., & Daya, M. (2014). Sensitivity, specificity, and sex differences in symptoms reported on the 13-item Acute Coronary Syndrome Checklist. *Journal of the American Heart Association, 3*, e000586.

4. Bergmann Lichtenstein, B. M. (2000). Emergence as a process of self-organizing: New assumptions and insights from the study of non-linear dynamic systems. *Journal of Organizational Change Management, 13*, 526–544.

5. Franklin, J. C., Ribeiro, J. D., Fox, K. R., Bentley, K. H., Kleiman, E. M., Huang, X., . . . & Nock, M. K. (2017). Risk factors for suicidal thoughts and behaviors: A meta-analysis of 50 years of research. *Psychological Bulletin, 143*, 187–232.

6. Simon, G. E., Rutter, C. M., Peterson, D., Oliver, M., Whiteside, U., Operskalski, B., & Ludman, E. J. (2013). Does response on the PHQ-9 Depression Questionnaire predict subsequent suicide attempt or suicide death? *Psychiatric Services, 64*, 1195–1202.

7. Anestis, M. D., & Green, B. A. (2015). The impact of varying levels of confidentiality on disclosure of suicidal thoughts in a sample of United States National Guard personnel. *Journal of Clinical Psychology, 71*, 1023–1030.

8. Vannoy, S. D., Andrews, B. K., Atkins, D. C., Dondanville, K. A., Young-McCaughan, S., Peterson, A. L., & STRONG STAR Consortium. (2017). Under reporting of suicide ideation in US Army population screening: An ongoing challenge. *Suicide and Life-Threatening Behavior, 47*, 723–728.

9. Mérelle, S., Foppen, E., Gilissen, R., Mokkenstorm, J., Cluitmans, R., & Van Ballegooijen, W. (2018). Characteristics associated with non-disclosure of suicidal ideation in adults. *International Journal of Environmental Research and Public Health, 15*, 943.

10. Richards, J. E., Whiteside, U., Ludman, E. J., Pabiniak, C., Kirlin, B., Hidalgo, R., & Simon, G. (2019). Understanding why patients may not report suicidal ideation at a health care visit prior to a suicide attempt: A qualitative study. *Psychiatric Services, 70*, 40–45.

11. Kleiman, E. M., Turner, B. J., Fedor, S., Beale, E. E., Huffman, J. C., & Nock, M. K. (2017). Examination of real-time fluctuations in suicidal ideation and its risk factors: Results from two ecological momentary assessment studies. *Journal of Abnormal Psychology, 126*, 726–738.

12. Kleiman, E. M., Turner, B. J., Fedor, S., Beale, E. E., Picard, R. W., Huffman, J. C., & Nock, M. K. (2018). Digital phenotyping of suicidal thoughts. *Depression and Anxiety, 35*, 601–608.

13. Bryan, C. J., & Rudd, M. D. (2018). Nonlinear change processes during psychotherapy characterize patients who have made multiple suicide attempts. *Suicide and Life-Threatening Behavior, 48*, 386–400.

14. Bryan, C. J., Rozek, D. C., Butner, J., & Rudd, M. D. (2019). Patterns of change in suicide ideation signal the recurrence of suicide attempts among high-risk psychiatric outpatients. *Behaviour Research and Therapy, 120*, 103392.

15. Franklin, J. (2018, June 11). Suicide prediction remains difficult despite decades of research. *Scientific American*. Available at https://www.scientificamerican.com/article/suicide-prediction-remains-difficult-despite-decades-of-research/

16. Gaynes, B. N., West, S. L., Ford, C. A., Frame, P., Klein, J., & Lohr, K. N. (2004). Screening for suicide risk in adults: A summary of the evidence for the US Preventive Services Task Force. *Annals of Internal Medicine, 140*, 822–835.

17. O'Connor, E., Gaynes, B., Burda, B., Williams, C., & Whitlock, E. (2013). *Screening for Suicide Risk in Primary Care: A Systematic Evidence Review for the US Preventive*

Service Task Force Agency for Healthcare Research and Quality. Evidence Synthesis No. 103. AHRQ Publication No. 13–05188-EF-1. Rockville, MD: Agency for Healthcare Research and Quality.

18. Mann, J. J., Apter, A., Bertolote, J., Beautrais, A., Currier, D., Haas, A., . . . & Mehlum, L. (2005). Suicide prevention strategies: A systematic review. *JAMA, 294,* 2064–2074.

19. Miller, I. W., Camargo, C. A., Arias, S. A., Sullivan, A. F., Allen, M. H., Goldstein, A. B., . . . & Boudreaux, E. D. (2017). Suicide prevention in an emergency department population: The ED-SAFE study. *JAMA Psychiatry, 74,* 563–570.

20. Bryan, C. J., Butner, J. E., Sinclair, S., Bryan, A. B. O., Hesse, C. M., & Rose, A. E. (2018). Predictors of emerging suicide death among military personnel on social media networks. *Suicide and Life-Threatening Behavior, 48,* 413–430.

21. Loveys, K., Crutchley, P., Wyatt, E., & Coppersmith, G. (2017). Small but mighty: Affective micropatterns for quantifying mental health from social media language. *Proceedings of the Fourth Workshop on Computational Linguistics and Clinical Psychology—From Linguistic Signal to Clinical Reality* (pp. 85–95). Stroudsburg, PA: Association for Computational Linguistics.

Chapter 4

1. Butner, J. E., Dyer, H. L., Malloy, T. S., & Kranz, L. V. (2014). Uncertainty in cost performance as a function of the cusp catastrophe in the NASA program performance management system. *Nonlinear Dynamics in Psychology and Life Sciences, 18,* 397–417.

2. Wyder, M., & De Leo, D. (2007). Behind impulsive suicide attempts: Indications from a community study. *Journal of Affective Disorders, 104,* 167–173.

3. Kessler, R. C., Borges, G., & Walters, E. E. (1999). Prevalence of and risk factors for lifetime suicide attempts in the National Comorbidity Survey. *Archives of General Psychiatry, 56,* 617–626.

4. Witte, T. K., Holm-Denoma, J. M., Zuromski, K. L., Gauthier, J. M., & Ruscio, J. (2017). Individuals at high risk for suicide are categorically distinct from those at low risk. *Psychological Assessment, 29,* 382–393.

5. Rufino, K. A., Marcus, D. K., Ellis, T. E., & Boccaccini, M. T. (2018). Further evidence that suicide risk is categorical: A taxometric analysis of data from an inpatient sample. *Psychological Assessment, 30,* 1541–1547.

6. Kessler, R. C., Warner, C. H., Ivany, C., Petukhova, M. V., Rose, S., Bromet, E. J., . . . & Fullerton, C. S. (2015). Predicting suicides after psychiatric hospitalization in US Army soldiers: The Army Study to Assess Risk and Resilience in Servicemembers (Army STARRS). *JAMA Psychiatry, 72,* 49–57.

7. Williams, C. L., Davidson, J. A., & Montgomery, I. (1980). Impulsive suicidal behavior. *Journal of Clinical Psychology, 36,* 90–94.

8. Simon, T. R., Swann, A. C., Powell, K. E., Potter, L. B., Kresnow, M. J., & O'Carroll, P. W. (2001). Characteristics of impulsive suicide attempts and attempters. *Suicide and Life-Threatening Behavior, 32 (Suppl 1),* 49–59.

9. Bryan, C. J., Garland, E. L., & Rudd, M. D. (2016). From impulse to action among military personnel hospitalized for suicide risk: Alcohol consumption and the reported transition from suicidal thought to behavior. *General Hospital Psychiatry, 41,* 13–19.

10. Millner, A. J., Lee, M. D., & Nock, M. K. (2017). Describing and measuring the pathway to suicide attempts: A preliminary study. *Suicide and Life-Threatening Behavior, 47*, 353–369.
11. Brown, G. K., Steer, R. A., Henriques, G. R., & Beck, A. T. (2005). The internal struggle between the wish to die and the wish to live: A risk factor for suicide. *American Journal of Psychiatry, 162*, 1977–1979.
12. Bryan, C. J., Rudd, M. D., Peterson, A. L., Young-McCaughan, S., & Wertenberger, E. G. (2016). The ebb and flow of the wish to live and the wish to die among suicidal military personnel. *Journal of Affective Disorders, 202*, 58–66.
13. Olfson, M., Wall, M., Wang, S., Crystal, S., Liu, S. M., Gerhard, T., & Blanco, C. (2016). Short-term suicide risk after psychiatric hospital discharge. *JAMA Psychiatry, 73*, 1119–1126.
14. Bryan, C. J., Rudd, M. D., & Wertenberger, E. (2013). Reasons for suicide attempts in a clinical sample of active duty soldiers. *Journal of Affective Disorders, 144*, 148–152.
15. Bryan, C. J., Rudd, M. D., & Wertenberger, E. (2016). Individual and environmental contingencies associated with multiple suicide attempts among US military personnel. *Psychiatry Research, 242*, 88–93.

Chapter 5

1. Battin, M. P. (2015). *The Ethics of Suicide: Historical Sources.* New York: Oxford University Press.
2. Franklin, J. C., Ribeiro, J. D., Fox, K. R., Bentley, K. H., Kleiman, E. M., Huang, X., . . . & Nock, M. K. (2017). Risk factors for suicidal thoughts and behaviors: A meta-analysis of 50 years of research. *Psychological Bulletin, 143*, 187–232.
3. Klonsky, E. D., Saffer, B. Y., & Bryan, C. J. (2018). Ideation-to-action theories of suicide: A conceptual and empirical update. *Current Opinion in Psychology, 22*, 38–43.
4. Bryan, C. J., Wood, D. S., May, A., Peterson, A. L., Wertenberger, E., & Rudd, M. D. (2018). Mechanisms of action contributing to reductions in suicide attempts following brief cognitive behavioral therapy for military personnel: A test of the interpersonal-psychological theory of suicide. *Archives of Suicide Research, 22*, 241–253.
5. Mischel, W., Ebbesen, E. B., & Raskoff Zeiss, A. (1972). Cognitive and attentional mechanisms in delay of gratification. *Journal of Personality and Social Psychology, 21*, 204–218.
6. Mischel, W., Shoda, Y., & Rodriguez, M. I. (1989). Delay of gratification in children. *Science, 244*, 933–938.
7. Ayduk, O., Mendoza-Denton, R., Mischel, W., Downey, G., Peake, P. K., & Rodriguez, M. (2000). Regulating the interpersonal self: Strategic self-regulation for coping with rejection sensitivity. *Journal of Personality and Social Psychology, 79*, 776–792.
8. Schlam, T. R., Wilson, N. L., Shoda, Y., Mischel, W., & Ayduk, O. (2013). Preschoolers' delay of gratification predicts their body mass 30 years later. *The Journal of Pediatrics, 162*, 90–93.
9. Shoda, Y., Mischel, W., & Peake, P. K. (1990). Predicting adolescent cognitive and self-regulatory competencies from preschool delay of gratification: Identifying diagnostic conditions. *Developmental Psychology, 26*, 978–986.
10. Mischel, W. (1958). Preference for delayed reinforcement: An experimental study of a cultural observation. *The Journal of Abnormal and Social Psychology, 56*, 57–61.

11. Mischel, W., & Ebbesen, E. B. (1970). Attention in delay of gratification. *Journal of Personality and Social Psychology, 16,* 329–337.

12. Casey, B. J., Somerville, L. H., Gotlib, I. H., Ayduk, O., Franklin, N. T., Askren, M. K., . . . & Glover, G. (2011). Behavioral and neural correlates of delay of gratification 40 years later. *Proceedings of the National Academy of Sciences, 108,* 14998–15003.

13. Mischel, W., & Grusec, J. (1967). Waiting for rewards and punishments: Effects of time and probability on choice. *Journal of Personality and Social Psychology, 5,* 24–31.

14. Watts, T. W., Duncan, G. J., & Quan, H. (2018). Revisiting the marshmallow test: A conceptual replication investigating links between early delay of gratification and later outcomes. *Psychological Science, 29,* 1159–1177.

15. Calarco, J. M. (2018, June 1). Why rich kids are so good at the marshmallow test. *The Atlantic.* Retrieved from https://www.theatlantic.com/family/archive/2018/06/marshmallow-test/561779/

16. Resnick, B. (2018, June 6). The "marshmallow test" said patience was a key to success; a new replication tells us s'more. *Vox.* Retrieved from https://www.vox.com/science-and-health/2018/6/6/17413000/marshmallow-test-replication-mischel-psychology

17. Dombrovski, A. Y., Szanto, K., Siegle, G. J., Wallace, M. L., Forman, S. D., Sahakian, B., . . . & Clark, L. (2011). Lethal forethought: Delayed reward discounting differentiates high-and low-lethality suicide attempts in old age. *Biological Psychiatry, 70,* 138–144.

18. Dombrovski, A. Y., Siegle, G. J., Szanto, K., Clark, L., Reynolds, C. F., & Aizenstein, H. (2012). The temptation of suicide: Striatal gray matter, discounting of delayed rewards, and suicide attempts in late-life depression. *Psychological Medicine, 42,* 1203–1215.

19. Wyart, M., Jaussent, I., Ritchie, K., Abbar, M., Jollant, F., & Courtet, P. (2016). Iowa Gambling Task performance in elderly persons with a lifetime history of suicidal acts. *American Journal of Geriatric Psychiatry, 24,* 399–406.

20. Jollant, F., Guillaume, S., Jaussent, I., Castelnau, D., Malafosse, A., & Courtet, P. (2007). Impaired decision-making in suicide attempters may increase the risk of problems in affective relationships. *Journal of Affective Disorders, 99,* 59–62.

21. Dombrovski, A. Y., Clark, L., Siegle, G. J., Butters, M. A., Ichikawa, N., Sahakian, B. J., & Szanto, K. (2010). Reward/punishment reversal learning in older suicide attempters. *American Journal of Psychiatry, 167,* 699–707.

22. Jollant, F., Lawrence, N. S., Giampietro, V., Brammer, M. J., Fullana, M. A., Drapier, D., . . . & Phillips, M. L. (2008). Orbitofrontal cortex response to angry faces in men with histories of suicide attempts. *American Journal of Psychiatry, 165,* 740–748.

23. Jollant, F., Lawrence, N. S., Olie, E., O'Daly, O., Malafosse, A., Courtet, P., & Phillips, M. L. (2010). Decreased activation of lateral orbitofrontal cortex during risky choices under uncertainty is associated with disadvantageous decision-making and suicidal behavior. *Neuroimage, 51,* 1275–1281.

24. Dombrovski, A. Y., Szanto, K., Clark, L., Reynolds, C. F., & Siegle, G. J. (2013). Reward signals, attempted suicide, and impulsivity in late-life depression. *JAMA Psychiatry, 70,* 1020–1030.

25. van den Bos, R., Homberg, J., & de Visser, L. (2013). A critical review of sex differences in decision-making tasks: Focus on the Iowa Gambling Task. *Behavioural Brain Research, 238,* 95–108.

26. Silverman, I. W. (2003). Gender differences in delay of gratification: A meta-analysis. *Sex Roles, 49,* 451–463.

Chapter 6

1. Helmuth, L. (2013, September 10). The disturbing, shameful history of childbirth deaths. *Slate*. Retrieved from http://www.slate.com/articles/health_and_science/science_of_longevity/2013/09/death_in_childbirth_doctors_increased_maternal_mortality_in_the_20th_century.html
2. Davis, R. (2015, January 12). The doctor who championed hand-washing and briefly saved lives. *NPR Morning Edition*. Retrieved from https://www.npr.org/sections/health-shots/2015/01/12/375663920/the-doctor-who-championed-hand-washing-and-saved-women-s-lives
3. World Health Organization. (2009). *WHO Guidelines on Hand Hygiene in Health Care*. Geneva, Austria: World Health Organization.
4. Semmelweis, I. (1983). *The Etiology, Concept, and Prophylaxis of Childbed Fever* (K. C. Carter, Trans.). Madison: The University of Wisconsin Press.
5. Fee, E., & Garofalo, M. E. (2010). Florence Nightingale and the Crimean War. *American Journal of Public Health, 100*, 1591.
6. Linehan, M. M. (1993). *Cognitive-Behavioral Treatment of Borderline Personality Disorder*. New York: Guilford Press.
7. Linehan, M. M., Armstrong, H. E., Suarez, A., Allmon, D., & Heard, H. L. (1991). Cognitive-behavioral treatment of chronically parasuicidal borderline patients. *Archives of General Psychiatry, 48*, 1060–1064.
8. Linehan, M. M., Comtois, K. A., Murray, A. M., Brown, M. Z., Gallop, R. J., Heard, H. L., & Lindenboim, N. (2006). Two-year randomized controlled trial and follow-up of dialectical behavior therapy vs therapy by experts for suicidal behaviors and borderline personality disorder. *Archives of General Psychiatry, 63*, 757–766.
9. Wenzel, A., Brown, G. K., & Beck, A. T. (2009). *Cognitive Therapy for Suicidal Patients: Scientific and Clinical Applications*. Washington, DC: American Psychological Association.
10. Brown, G. K., Ten Have, T., Henriques, G. R., Xie, S. X., Hollander, J. E., & Beck, A. T. (2005). Cognitive therapy for the prevention of suicide attempts: A randomized controlled trial. *JAMA, 294*, 563–570.
11. Bryan, C. J., & Rudd, M. D. (2018). *Brief Cognitive Behavioral Therapy for Suicide Prevention*. New York: Guilford Publications.
12. Rudd, M. D., Bryan, C. J., Wertenberger, E., Peterson, A. L., Young-McCaughon, S., Mintz, J., & Bruce, T. O. (2015). Brief cognitive behavioral therapy effects on post-treatment suicide attempts in a military sample: Results of a 2-year randomized clinical trial. *American Journal of Psychiatry, 172*, 441–449.
13. Sinyor, M., Williams, M., Mitchell, R., Zaheer, R., Bryan, C.J., Schaffer, A., . . ., & Selchen, S. (2020). Cognitive behavioral therapy for suicide prevention in youth admitted to hospital following an episode of self-harm: A pilot randomized controlled trial. *Journal of Affective Disorders, 266*, 686–694.
14. Rudd, M. D., Joiner Jr, T. E., & Rajab, M. H. (2001). *Treating Suicidal Behavior: An Effective, Time-Limited Approach*. New York: Guilford Press.
15. Bryan, C. J., Mintz, J., Clemans, T. A., Leeson, B., Burch, T. S., Williams, S. R., . . . & Rudd, M. D. (2017). Effect of crisis response planning vs. contracts for safety on suicide risk in US Army soldiers: A randomized clinical trial. *Journal of Affective Disorders, 212*, 64–72.

16. Michel, K., & Gysin-Maillart, A. (2015). *ASSIP: Attempted Suicide Short Intervention Program: A Manual for Clinicians*. Ashland, OH: Hogrefe Publishing.

17. Gysin-Maillart, A., Schwab, S., Soravia, L., Megert, M., & Michel, K. (2016). A novel brief therapy for patients who attempt suicide: A 24-months follow-up randomized controlled study of the Attempted Suicide Short Intervention Program (ASSIP). *PLOS Medicine, 13*(3), e1001968.

18. Bateman, A., & Fonagy, P. (2008). 8-year follow-up of patients treated for border-line personality disorder: Mentalization-based treatment versus treatment as usual. *American Journal of Psychiatry, 165*, 631–638.

19. Jobes, D. A. (2016). *Managing Suicidal Risk: A Collaborative Approach* (2nd ed.). New York: Guilford Press.

20. Jobes, D.A. (2012). The Collaborative Assessment and Management of Suicidality (CAMS): An evolving evidence-based clinical approach to suicidal risk. *Suicide and Life-Threatening Behavior, 42*, 640–653.

21. Tarrier, N., Taylor, K., & Gooding, P. (2008). Cognitive-behavioral interventions to re-duce suicide behavior: A systematic review and meta-analysis. *Behavior Modification, 32*, 77–108.

22. Bryan, C. J., & Rozek, D. C. (2018). Suicide prevention in the military: A mechanistic perspective. *Current Opinion in Psychology, 22*, 27–32.

23. Bryan, C. J., Clemans, T. A., Hernandez, A. M., Mintz, J., Peterson, A. L., Yarvis, J. S., . . . & STRONG STAR Consortium. (2016). Evaluating potential iatrogenic suicide risk in trauma-focused group cognitive behavioral therapy for the treatment of PTSD in active duty military personnel. *Depression and Anxiety, 33*, 549–557.

24. Gradus, J. L., Suvak, M. K., Wisco, B. E., Marx, B. P., & Resick, P. A. (2013). Treatment of posttraumatic stress disorder reduces suicidal ideation. *Depression and Anxiety, 30*, 1046–1053.

25. Trockel, M., Karlin, B. E., Taylor, C. B., Brown, G. K., & Manber, R. (2015). Effects of cognitive behavioral therapy for insomnia on suicidal ideation in veterans. *Sleep, 38*, 259–265.

26. Bruce, M. L., Ten Have, T. R., Reynolds III, C. F., Katz, I. I., Schulberg, H. C., Mulsant, B. H., . . . & Alexopoulos, G. S. (2004). Reducing suicidal ideation and depressive symptoms in depressed older primary care patients: A randomized controlled trial. *JAMA, 291*, 1081–1091.

27. Linehan, M. M., Korslund, K. E., Harned, M. S., Gallop, R. J., Lungu, A., Neacsiu, A. D., . . . & Murray-Gregory, A. M. (2015). Dialectical behavior therapy for high suicide risk in individuals with borderline personality disorder: A randomized clinical trial and component analysis. *JAMA Psychiatry, 72*, 475–482.

28. Menon, V. (2011). Large-scale brain networks and psychopathology: A unifying triple network model. *Trends in Cognitive Sciences, 15*, 483–506.

29. Zhang, S., Chen, J. M., Kuang, L., Cao, J., Zhang, H., Ai, M., . . . & Fang, W. D. (2016). Association between abnormal default mode network activity and suicidality in de-pressed adolescents. *BMC Psychiatry, 16*, 337.

30. Martin, P. C., Zimmer, T. J., & Pan, L. A. (2015). Magnetic resonance imaging markers of suicide attempt and suicide risk in adolescents. *CNS Spectrums, 20*, 355–358.

31. Ordaz, S. J., Goyer, M. S., Ho, T. C., Singh, M. K., & Gotlib, I. H. (2018). Network basis of suicidal ideation in depressed adolescents. *Journal of Affective Disorders, 226*, 92–99.

32. Doll, A., Sorg, C., Manoliu, A., Meng, C., Wöller, A., Förstl, H., . . . & Riedl, V. (2013). Shifted intrinsic connectivity of central executive and salience network in borderline personality disorder. *Frontiers in Human Neuroscience, 7,* 727.

33. Davidson, R. J., Jackson, D. C., & Kalin, N. H. (2000). Emotion, plasticity, context, and regulation: Perspectives from affective neuroscience. *Psychological Bulletin, 126,* 890–909.

34. Jollant, F., Lawrence, N. S., Giampietro, V., Brammer, M. J., Fullana, M. A., Drapier, D., . . . & Phillips, M. L. (2008). Orbitofrontal cortex response to angry faces in men with histories of suicide attempts. *American Journal of Psychiatry, 165,* 740–748.

35. Jollant, F., Lawrence, N. S., Olie, E., O'Daly, O., Malafosse, A., Courtet, P., & Phillips, M. L. (2010). Decreased activation of lateral orbitofrontal cortex during risky choices under uncertainty is associated with disadvantageous decision-making and suicidal behavior. *Neuroimage, 51,* 1275–1281.

36. Dombrovski, A. Y., Szanto, K., Clark, L., Reynolds, C. F., & Siegle, G. J. (2013). Reward signals, attempted suicide, and impulsivity in late-life depression. *JAMA Psychiatry, 70,* 1020–1030.

37. Pan, L. A., Hassel, S., Segreti, A. M., Nau, S. A., Brent, D. A., & Phillips, M. L. (2013). Differential patterns of activity and functional connectivity in emotion processing neural circuitry to angry and happy faces in adolescents with and without suicide attempt. *Psychological Medicine, 43,* 2129–2142.

38. Pan, L., Segreti, A., Almeida, J., Jollant, F., Lawrence, N., Brent, D., & Phillips, M. (2013). Preserved hippocampal function during learning in the context of risk in adolescent suicide attempt. *Psychiatry Research: Neuroimaging, 211,* 112–118.

39. Davidson, R. J., Marshall, J. R., Tomarken, A. J., & Henriques, J. B. (2000). While a phobic waits: Regional brain electrical and autonomic activity in social phobics during anticipation of public speaking. *Biological Psychiatry, 47,* 85–95.

40. Abdallah, C. G., Averill, C. L., Ramage, A. E., Averill, L. A., Alkin, E., Nemati, S., . . . & Peterson, A. L. (2019). Reduced salience and enhanced central executive connectivity following PTSD treatment. *Chronic Stress, 3,* 2470547019838971.

41. Mann, J. J. (2003). Neurobiology of suicidal behaviour. *Nature Reviews Neuroscience, 4,* 819–828.

42. Rudd, M. D., Mandrusiak, M., & Joiner, T. E. (2006). The case against no-suicide contracts: The commitment to treatment statement as a practice alternative. *Journal of Clinical Psychology, 62,* 243–251.

43. National Action Alliance for Suicide Prevention (2018). *Recommended Standard Care for People with Suicide Risk: Making Health Care Suicide Safe.* Washington, DC: Education Development Center.

44. The Joint Commission. (2016). *Sentinel Event Alert: Detecting and Treating Suicide Ideation in All Settings.* Retrieved from https://www.jointcommission.org/assets/1/18/SEA_56_Suicide.pdf

45. Schmitz Jr, W. M., Allen, M. H., Feldman, B. N., Gutin, N. J., Jahn, D. R., Kleespies, P. M., . . . & Simpson, S. (2012). Preventing suicide through improved training in suicide risk assessment and care: An American Association of Suicidology Task Force report addressing serious gaps in US mental health training. *Suicide and Life-Threatening Behavior, 42,* 292–304.

46. Gamarra, J. M., Luciano, M. T., Gradus, J. L., & Stirman, S. W. (2015). Assessing variability and implementation fidelity of suicide prevention safety planning in a regional VA healthcare system. *Crisis, 36,* 433–439.

47. Green, J. D., Kearns, J. C., Rosen, R. C., Keane, T. M., & Marx, B. P. (2018). Evaluating the effectiveness of safety plans for military veterans: Do safety plans tailored to veteran characteristics decrease suicide risk? *Behavior Therapy, 49*, 931–938.
48. Wharff, E. A., Ross, A. M., & Lambert, S. (2014). Field note—developing suicide risk assessment training for hospital social workers: An academic-community partnership. *Journal of Social Work Education, 50*, 184–190.
49. Substance Abuse and Mental Health Service Administration. (2018). *Key Substance Use and Mental Health Indicators in the United States: Results from the 2017 National Survey on Drug Use and Health (HHS Publication No. SMA 18-5068, NSDUH Series H-53)*. Rockville, MD: Center for Behavioral Health Statistics and Quality, Substance Abuse and Mental Health Services Administration.
50. Bernecker, S. L., Zuromski, K. L., Curry, J. C., Kim, J. J., Gutierrez, P. M., Joiner T. E., . . ., & Bryan, C. J. (in press). An economic evaluation of brief cognitive behavioral therapy vs treatment as usual for suicidal U.S. Army Soldiers. *JAMA Psychiatry, 77*, 256–264.
51. Kessler, R. C., Berglund, P., Borges, G., Nock, M., & Wang, P. S. (2005). Trends in suicide ideation, plans, gestures, and attempts in the United States, 1990–1992 to 2001–2003. *JAMA Psychiatry, 293*, 2487–2495.

Chapter 7

1. Davis, S. C., & Boundy, R. G. (2019). *Transportation Energy Data Book: Edition 37.1*. Oak Ridge, TN: Oak Ridge National Laboratory.
2. Fairfield, H. (2012, September 17). Driving Safety, in fits and starts. *The New York Times*. Retrieved from https://archive.nytimes.com/www.nytimes.com/interactive/2012/09/17/science/driving-safety-in-fits-and-starts.html
3. National Safety Council. (2019). *Car Crash Deaths and Rates*. Retrieved from https://injuryfacts.nsc.org/motor-vehicle/historical-fatality-trends/deaths-and-rates/
4. World Health Organization. (2006). *Road Traffic Injury Prevention Training Manual*. New Delhi, India: Indian Institute of Technology Delhi.
5. U.S. Department of Transportation. (2008). *How States Achieve High Seat Belt Use Rates*. Springfield, VA: National Technical Information Service.
6. Harvard University. (2019). *Harvard Alcohol Project*. Retrieved from https://www.hsph.harvard.edu/chc/harvard-alcohol-project/
7. National Institutes of Health. (2010). *Fact Sheet: Alcohol-Related Traffic Deaths*. Retrieved from https://report.nih.gov/nihfactsheets/Pdfs/AlcoholRelatedTrafficDeaths(NIAAA).pdf
8. National Highway Traffic Safety Administration (2017). *USDOT Releases 2016 Fatal Traffic Crash Data*. Retrieved from https://www.nhtsa.gov/press-releases/usdot-releases-2016-fatal-traffic-crash-data
9. Mann, J. J., Apter, A., Bertolote, J., Beautrais, A., Currier, D., Haas, A., . . . & Mehlum, L. (2005). Suicide prevention strategies: A systematic review. *JAMA, 294*, 2064–2074.
10. Kreitman, N. (1976). The coal gas story: United Kingdom suicide rates, 1960–71. *British Journal of Epidemiology and Community Health, 30*, 86–93.
11. Gunnell, D., Fernando, R., Hewagama, M., Priyangika, W. D., Konradsen, F., & Eddleston, M. (2007). The impact of pesticide regulations on suicide in Sri Lanka. *International Journal of Epidemiology, 36*, 1235–1242.

12. Bowles, J. R. (1995). An example of a suicide prevention program in a developing country. In R. F. W. Diekstra, W. Gulbinat, I. Kienhorst, & D. de Leo (Eds.), *Preventive Strategies on Suicide* (pp. 173–206). Leiden, The Netherlands: E. J. Brill.

13. Hawton, K. (2002). United Kingdom legislation on pack sizes of analgesics: Background, rationale, and effects on suicide and deliberate self-harm. *Suicide and Life-Threatening Behavior, 32,* 223–229.

14. Oliver, R. G., & Hetzel, B. S. (1972). Rise and fall of suicide rates in Australia: Relation to sedative availability. *Medical Journal of Australia, 2,* 919–923.

15. Nordentoft, M., Qin, P., Helweg-Larsen, K., & Juel, K. (2007). Restrictions in means for suicide: An effective tool in preventing suicide: The Danish experience. *Suicide and Life-Threatening Behavior, 37,* 688–697.

16. Pirkis, J., Spittal, M. J., Cox, G., Robinson, J., Cheung, Y. T. D., & Studdert, D. (2013). The effectiveness of structural interventions at suicide hotspots: A meta-analysis. *International Journal of Epidemiology, 42,* 541–548.

17. Bennewith, O., Nowers, M., & Gunnell, D. (2007). Effect of barriers on the Clifton suspension bridge, England, on local patterns of suicide: Implications for prevention. *British Journal of Psychiatry, 190,* 266–267.

18. O'Carroll, P. W., Silverman, M. M., & Berman, A. L. (1994). Community suicide prevention: The effectiveness of bridge barriers. *Suicide and Life-Threatening Behavior, 24,* 89–99.

19. Pelletier, A. R. (2007). Preventing suicide by jumping: The effect of a bridge safety fence. *Injury Prevention, 13,* 57–59.

20. Beautrais, A. L., Gibb, S. J., Fergusson, D. M., Horwood, L. J., & Larkin, G. L. (2009). Removing bridge barriers stimulates suicides: An unfortunate natural experiment. *Australian & New Zealand Journal of Psychiatry, 43,* 495–497.

21. Elnour, A. A., & Harrison, J. (2008). Lethality of suicide methods. *Injury Prevention, 14,* 39–45.

22. Centers for Disease Control and Prevention. (n.d.). *Web-Based Injury Statistics Query and Reporting System (WISQARS) Fatal Injury Data.* Retrieved from https://www.cdc.gov/injury/wisqars.fatal.html

23. Loftin, C., McDowall, D., Wiersema, B., & Cottey, T. J. (1991). Effects of restrictive licensing of handguns on homicide and suicide in the District of Columbia. *New England Journal of Medicine, 325,* 1615–1620.

24. Lubin, G., Werbeloff, N., Halperin, D., Shmushkevitch, M., Weiser, M., & Knobler, H. Y. (2010). Decrease in suicide rates after a change of policy reducing access to firearms in adolescents: A naturalistic epidemiological study. *Suicide and Life-Threatening Behavior, 40,* 421–424.

25. Anestis, M. D., & Anestis, J. C. (2015). Suicide rates and state laws regulating access and exposure to handguns. *American Journal of Public Health, 105,* 2049–2058.

26. Cummings, P., Grossman, D. C., Rivara, F. P., & Koepsell, T. D. (1997). State gun safe storage laws and child mortality due to firearms. *JAMA, 278,* 1084–1086.

27. Grossman, D. C., Mueller, B. A., Riedy, C., Dowd, M. D., Villaveces, A., Prodzinski, J., . . . & Harruff, R. (2005). Gun storage practices and risk of youth suicide and unintentional firearm injuries. *JAMA, 293,* 707–714.

28. Shenassa, E. D., Rogers, M. L., Spalding, K. L., & Roberts, M. B. (2004). Safer storage of firearms at home and risk of suicide: A study of protective factors in a nationally representative sample. *Journal of Epidemiology & Community Health, 58,* 841–848.

29. Brent, D. A., Perper, J. A., Moritz, G., Baugher, M., Schweers, J., & Roth, C. (1993). Firearms and adolescent suicide: A community case-control study. *American Journal of Diseases of Children, 147*, 1066–1071.

30. Kellermann, A. L., Rivara, F. P., Rushforth, N. B., Banton, J. G., Reay, D. T., Francisco, J. T., . . . & Somes, G. (1993). Gun ownership as a risk factor for homicide in the home. *New England Journal of Medicine, 329*, 1084–1091.

31. Owens, D., Horrocks, J., & House, A. (2002). Fatal and non-fatal repetition of self-harm: Systematic review. *The British Journal of Psychiatry, 181*, 193–199.

32. Khazem, L. R., Houtsma, C., Gratz, K. L., Tull, M. T., Green, B. A., & Anestis, M. D. (2015). Firearms matter: The moderating role of firearm storage in the association between current suicidal ideation and likelihood of future suicide attempts among United States military personnel. *Military Psychology, 28*, 25–33.

33. Marino, E., Wolsko, C., Keys, S., & Wilcox, H. (2018). Addressing the cultural challenges of firearm restriction in suicide prevention: A test of public health messaging to protect those at risk. *Archives of Suicide Research, 22*, 394–404.

Chapter 8

1. Gertner, A. K., Rotter, J. S., & Shafer, P. R. (2019). Association between state minimum wages and suicide rates in the US. *American Journal of Preventive Medicine, 56*, 648–654.

2. Tondo, L., Albert, M. J., & Baldessarini, R. J. (2006). Suicide rates in relation to health care access in the United States: An ecological study. *The Journal of Clinical Psychiatry, 67*, 517–523.

3. Tondo, M. (2013). The impact of mental health insurance laws on state suicide rates. *Health Economics, 22*, 73–88.

4. Wang, P. S., Lane, M., Olfson, M., Pincus, H. A., Wells, K. B., & Kessler, R. C. (2005). Twelve-month use of mental health services in the United States: Results from the National Comorbidity Survey Replication. *Archives of General Psychiatry, 62*, 629–640.

5. Bakian, A. V., Huber, R. S., Coon, H., Gray, D., Wilson, P., McMahon, W. M., & Renshaw, P. F. (2015). Acute air pollution exposure and risk of suicide completion. *American Journal of Epidemiology, 181*, 295–303.

6. Resick, P. A., Monson, C. M., & Chard, K. M. (2016). *Cognitive Processing Therapy for PTSD: A Comprehensive Manual*. New York: Guilford Publications.

7. Department of Veterans Affairs and Department of Defense. (2017). *VA/DoD Clinical Practice Guideline for the Management of Posttraumatic Stress Disorder and Acute Stress Disorder*. Washington, DC: Department of Veterans Affairs and Department of Defense.

8. Berg, A. O., Breslau, N., Goodman, S. N., Lezak, M., Matchar, D., Mellman, T. A., . . . & Geller, A. (2007). *Treatment of PTSD: An Assessment of the Evidence*. Washington, DC: National Academies Press.

9. Watts, B. V., Schnurr, P. P., Mayo, L., Young-Xu, Y., Weeks, W. B., & Friedman, M. J. (2013). Meta-analysis of the efficacy of treatments for posttraumatic stress disorder. *Journal of Clinical Psychiatry, 74*, e541–e550.

10. Gilboa-Schechtman, E., & Foa, E. B. (2001). Patterns of recovery from trauma: The use of intraindividual analysis. *Journal of Abnormal Psychology, 110*, 392–400.

11. O'Donnell, M. L., Elliott, P., Lau, W., & Creamer, M. (2007). PTSD symptom trajectories: From early to chronic response. *Behaviour Research and Therapy, 45*, 601–606.

12. Galatzer-Levy, I. R., Ankri, Y., Freedman, S., Israeli-Shalev, Y., Roitman, P., Gilad, M., & Shalev, A. Y. (2013). Early PTSD symptom trajectories: Persistence, recovery, and response to treatment: Results from the Jerusalem Trauma Outreach and Prevention Study (J-TOPS). *PloS One, 8*, e70084.

13. Pietrzak, R. H., Feder, A., Singh, R., Schechter, C. B., Bromet, E. J., Katz, C. L., . . . & Harrison, D. (2014). Trajectories of PTSD risk and resilience in World Trade Center responders: An 8-year prospective cohort study. *Psychological Medicine, 44*, 205–219.

14. Bryan, C. J., Leifker, F. R., Rozek, D. C., Bryan, A. O., Reynolds, M. L., Oakey, D. N., & Roberge, E. (2018). Examining the effectiveness of an intensive, 2-week treatment program for military personnel and veterans with PTSD: Results of a pilot, open-label, prospective cohort trial. *Journal of Clinical Psychology, 74*, 2070–2081.

15. Menon, V. (2011). Large-scale brain networks and psychopathology: A unifying triple network model. *Trends in Cognitive Sciences, 15*, 483–506.

16. Mann, J. J. (2003). Neurobiology of suicidal behaviour. *Nature Reviews Neuroscience, 4*, 819–828.

17. Abdallah, C. G., Averill, C. L., Ramage, A. E., Averill, L. A., Alkin, E., Nemati, S., . . . & Peterson, A. L. (2019). Reduced salience and enhanced central executive connectivity following PTSD treatment. *Chronic Stress, 3*, 2470547019838971.

18. Harik, J. M., Grubbs, K. G., & Schnurr, P. P. (2016, November). Using graphics to communicate information about PTSD treatment effectiveness to patients. In J. L. Hamblen (Chair), *Enhancing the Quality of Online Information to Support PTSD Treatment Engagement*. Symposium presented at the 30th annual meeting of the International Society for Traumatic Stress Studies, Dallas, TX.

19. Resick, P. A., Williams, L. F., Suvak, M. K., Monson, C. M., & Gradus, J. L. (2012). Long-term outcomes of cognitive–behavioral treatments for posttraumatic stress disorder among female rape survivors. *Journal of Consulting and Clinical Psychology, 80*, 201–210.

20. Bryan, C. J., Clemans, T. A., Hernandez, A. M., Mintz, J., Peterson, A. L., Yarvis, J. S., . . . & STRONG STAR Consortium. (2016). Evaluating potential iatrogenic suicide risk in trauma-focused group cognitive behavioral therapy for the treatment of PTSD in active duty military personnel. *Depression and Anxiety, 33*, 549–557.

21. Gradus, J. L., Suvak, M. K., Wisco, B. E., Marx, B. P., & Resick, P. A. (2013). Treatment of posttraumatic stress disorder reduces suicidal ideation. *Depression and Anxiety, 30*, 1046–1053.

22. Rudd, M. D., Bryan, C. J., Wertenberger, E. G., Peterson, A. L., Young-McCaughan, S., Mintz, J., . . . & Wilkinson, E. (2015). Brief cognitive-behavioral therapy effects on post-treatment suicide attempts in a military sample: Results of a randomized clinical trial with 2-year follow-up. *American Journal of Psychiatry, 172*, 441–449.

23. Bryan, C. J., Rudd, M. D., Peterson, A. L., Young-McCaughan, S., & Wertenberger, E. G. (2016). The ebb and flow of the wish to live and the wish to die among suicidal military personnel. *Journal of Affective Disorders, 202*, 58–66.

24. Bryan, C. J., & Rudd, M. D. (2018). *Brief Cognitive-Behavioral Therapy for Suicide Prevention*. New York: Guilford Publications.

25. Arie, M., Apter, A., Orbach, I., Yefet, Y., & Zalzman, G. (2008). Autobiographical memory, interpersonal problem solving, and suicidal behavior in adolescent inpatients. *Comprehensive Psychiatry, 49*, 22–29.

26. Pollock, L. R., & Williams, J. M. G. (2001). Effective problem solving in suicide attempters depends on specific autobiographical recall. *Suicide and Life-Threatening Behavior, 31,* 386–396.

27. Rozek, D. C., Keane, C., Sippel, L. M., Stein, J. Y., Rollo-Carlson, C., & Bryan, C. J. (2019). Short-term effects of crisis response planning on optimism in a US Army sample. *Early Intervention in Psychiatry, 13,* 682–685.

28. Bryan, C. J., Mintz, J., Clemans, T. A., Burch, T. S., Leeson, B., Williams, S., & Rudd, M. D. (2017). Effect of crisis response planning on patient mood and clinician decision making: A clinical trial with suicidal US soldiers. *Psychiatric Services, 69,* 108–111.

29. Bryan, C. J., Bryan, A. O., Rozek, D. C., & Leifker, R. R. (2019). *Meaning in Life Drives Reductions in Suicide Risk Among Acutely Suicidal Soldiers Receiving a Crisis Response Plan.* Manuscript submitted for publication.

30. Linehan, M. M., Goodstein, J. L., Nielsen, S. L., & Chiles, J. A. (1983). Reasons for staying alive when you are thinking of killing yourself: The Reasons for Living Inventory. *Journal of Consulting and Clinical Psychology, 51,* 276–286.

31. Osman, A., Downs, W. R., Kopper, B. A., Barrios, F. X., Baker, M. T., Osman, J. R., . . . & Linehan, M. M. (1998). The Reasons for Living Inventory for Adolescents (RFL-A): Development and psychometric properties. *Journal of Clinical Psychology, 54,* 1063–1078.

32. Osman, A., Gifford, J., Jones, T., Lickiss, L., Osman, J., & Wenzel, R. (1993). Psychometric evaluation of the Reasons for Living Inventory. *Psychological Assessment, 5,* 154–158.

33. Ivanoff, A., Jang, S. J., Smyth, N. J., & Linehan, M. M. (1994). Fewer reasons for staying alive when you are thinking of killing yourself: The Brief Reasons for Living Inventory. *Journal of Psychopathology and Behavioral Assessment, 16,* 1–13.

34. Bryan, C. J., Oakey, D. N., & Harris, J. A. (2018). Reasons for living among US Army personnel thinking about suicide. *Cognitive Therapy and Research, 42,* 758–768.

35. Bryan, C. J., Rudd, M. D., & Wertenberger, E. (2013). Reasons for suicide attempts in a clinical sample of active duty soldiers. *Journal of Affective Disorders, 144,* 148–152.

36. Bryan, C. J., Rudd, M. D., & Wertenberger, E. (2016). Individual and environmental contingencies associated with multiple suicide attempts among US military personnel. *Psychiatry Research, 242,* 88–93.

37. Bryan, C. J., May, A. M., & Harris, J. (2018). Examining emotion relief motives as a facilitator of the transition from suicidal thought to first suicide attempt among active duty soldiers. *Psychological Services, 16,* 293–301.

38. Jobes, D. A. (2016). *Managing Suicidal Risk: A Collaborative Approach* (2nd ed.). New York: Guilford Publications.

39. Substance Abuse and Mental Health Service Administration. (2018). *Key Substance Use and Mental Health Indicators in the United States: Results from the 2017 National Survey on Drug Use and Health (HHS Publication No. SMA 18-5068, NSDUH Series H-53).* Rockville, MD: Center for Behavioral Health Statistics and Quality, Substance Abuse and Mental Health Services Administration.

40. Fowler, J. H., & Christakis, N. A. (2008). Dynamic spread of happiness in a large social network: Longitudinal analysis over 20 years in the Framingham Heart Study. *British Medical Journal, 337,* a2338.

41. Bryan, C. J., Bryan, A. O., Rugo, K. F., Hinkson, K. D., & Leifker, F. R. (2019). Happiness, meaning in life, and PTSD symptoms among National Guard personnel: A multilevel analysis. *Journal of Happiness Studies, 21,* 1251–1264.

42. Bryan, C. J., Elder, W. B., McNaughton-Cassill, M., Osman, A., Hernandez, A. M., & Allison, S. (2013). Meaning in life, emotional distress, suicidal ideation, and life functioning in an active duty military sample. *The Journal of Positive Psychology, 8*, 444–452.

43. Kleiman, E. M., & Beaver, J. K. (2013). A meaningful life is worth living: Meaning in life as a suicide resiliency factor. *Psychiatry Research, 210*, 934–939.

44. Lambert, N. M., Stillman, T. F., Hicks, J. A., Kamble, S., Baumeister, R. F., & Fincham, F. D. (2013). To belong is to matter: Sense of belonging enhances meaning in life. *Personality and Social Psychology Bulletin, 39*, 1418–1427.

45. Diener, E. (2000). Subjective well-being: The science of happiness and a proposal for a national index. *American Psychologist, 55*, 34–43.

46. Coley, R. L., & Brunson, L. (1998). Fertile ground for community: Inner-city neighborhood common spaces. *American Journal of Community Psychology, 26*, 823–851.

47. Huffman, J. C., DuBois, C. M., Healy, B. C., Boehm, J. K., Kashdan, T. B., Celano, C. M., . . . & Lyubomirsky, S. (2014). Feasibility and utility of positive psychology exercises for suicidal inpatients. *General Hospital Psychiatry, 36*, 88–94.

48. Lyubomirsky, S., Dickerhoof, R., Boehm, J. K., & Sheldon, K. M. (2011). Becoming happier takes both a will and a proper way: An experimental longitudinal intervention to boost well-being. *Emotion, 11*, 391–402.

Index